APD
38

D1881013

FUNDAMENTALS OF NURSING

FUNDAMENTALS
OF
NURSING

Sanjeev Singh

genNEXT Publication

Fundamentals of Nursing

Rs. 890

© Sanjeev Singh

ISBN: 978-81-908675-2-8

All rights reserved. No Part of this book may be reproduced in any manner without written permission.

Published in 2010 in India by
Gennext Publication
23 Main Ansari Road, Darya Ganj,
New Delhi-110002
E-Mail:GenNextpublication@hotmail.com
Phone: 23282060

Printed at: Singhal Print Media, Delhi

Contents

Preface

In the upcoming decade, more than ever before, nurses will be expected to provide evidence-based care for patients. This approach requires us to have a sound working knowledge of strong clinical foundation. As reforms emerge, nursing's role will be a central one in shaping the policies, structures, and practices to advance access as a national objective. Looking forward, the theme of this text collaboration for optimal health is quite relevant with the revised syllabus of the Nursing Council of India. The rapid expansion of managed care, to date the major trend in health care reform, makes it so. Managed care, while on the one hand fostering interdisciplinary professional collaboration with its pressures for cost-containment, also brings economic constraints to bear on patient-provider collaboration, often with controversial results.

The environment of health care continues to grow more challenging day by day which means that nursing education will be under constant pressure to align its curricula with the driving forces of change. As a new era opens, the fast-paced scientific advances and ever-changing technology of the 20th Century will persist as important characteristics of the health care environment, as will the provider specialization they promote, delivery system reforms notwithstanding.

At the same time that the information in these areas of nursing is increasing, less time is available in nursing programs to cover it. Students experience difûculty reading all of the material available in the market. So I here put my efforts and experience to capsule the whole syllabus of Nursing in this book including all the topics in a precise but comprehensible manner. Undersigned is confident enough that this book will be a handy tool in the students of nursing. Your sincere feedback always encourage me to improve my way of presentation. Reader's suggestions and comments are always welcome.

1

Introduction

Health is one of our most cherished possessions. The preservation of health is met through the gratification of our fundamental human needs. Realizing the fundamental needs of people, hence, is essential for the practical nurse in planning for and meeting the needs of the patient.

CONCEPT OF HEALTH

A person's notion of health is a very personal thing. One individual may consider himself to be healthy each time he is not physically ill, while another may consider himself to be fit only when he is emotionally and physically "at his best." A person's belief of health is determined by a number of different components or experiences, such as family background, self-notion, religion, past experiences, and socioeconomic status. It is significant that you, as a practical nurse, keep this in mind when dealing with your patient's, as well as your own, feelings and interactions.

For intentions of this course, we will define health as a state of total physical, mental, and social well-being, not merely the lack of disease or infirmity.

Though the absence of disease and illness is, by anyone's definition, essential to good health, it is, by no means, the only component. Total health includes all of the following aspects as well:

- Social health: A sense of duty for the health and welfare of others.
- Mental health: A mind that grows, reasons, and adjusts to life situations.
- Emotional health: Feelings and actions that bring one satisfaction.
- Spiritual health: Inner peace and security in one's spiritual faith.

THE HEALTH-ILLNESS CONTINUUM

The individual's state of health is one of continuous change. He moves back and forth from health to illness and back to health again. His circumstance is rarely constant. He may wake up feeling great, develop a headache mid-morning, and feel fine again by noon. The health-illness continuum shows this process of change, in which the person goes through various states of health and illness (ranging from extremely good health to death) that fluctuate throughout his life.

As we previously stated, health, just as life itself, is a process of continuous change. And we must continuously adapt to these changes in our lives in order to maintain good health and well-being. It is our adaptation or response to that change, rather than the change itself, that affects our health. For instance, two students just found out about a big test tomorrow, for which they are completely unprepared. One student responds to this stressful situation (stressor) by going home, getting his books out, and starting to study.

The other student breaks out into a sweat, and spends most of the evening fretting over this outrage and imagining what will happen to him if he doesn't pass the test. No doubt, this student is doing more damage to his health than is his friend. And, considering the time and energy he is expending on worrying (and not studying), he may experience even more stress when they receive their grades.

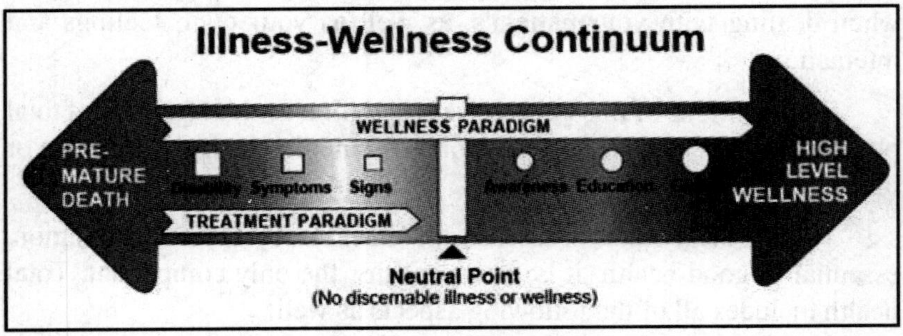

Fig. Health-Illness Continuum

Adaptation and effective functioning, even in the presence of chronic disease, can be considered a state of wellness. An individual may be in perfect physical condition, but feel too tired and "blue" to go to work, while his co-worker, a diabetic, is at work, functioning fully and accomplishing his job.

FACTORS INFLUENCING HEALTH

The person's state of health is determined by the ability to adapt to changes in the following dimensions:

- Developmental: changes in a person's behaviour and ability, which are associated with increasing age.
- Psychosocial: the development of the personality, social attitudes, and skills.
- Cultural: changes in or development of beliefs and values held by the person's family or culture.
- Physiological: changes in body function.

CAUSES AND RISK FACTORS FOR DEVELOPING ILLNESS

How illness is explained often varies radically from culture to culture. Likewise, the methods considered acceptable for curing illness in one culture may be rejected by another. These differences can be broadly generalized in terms of two explanatory traditions: naturalistic and personalistic.

The World now mostly relies on a naturalistic explanation of illness. This medical tradition had its beginnings in ancient Greece, especially with the ideas of Hippocrates in the 4th and 5th centuries B.C. However, it didn't begin to take its modern form until the 16th century A.D.

The naturalistic explanation assumes that illness is only due to impersonal, mechanistic causes in nature that can be potentially understood and cured by the application of the scientific method of discovery. Common causes of illness accepted in naturalistic medical systems include:

- Organic breakdown or deterioration (e.g., tooth decay, heart failure, senility)
- Obstruction (e.g., kidney stones, arterial blockage due to plaque build-up)
- Injury (e.g., broken bones, bullet wounds)
- Imbalance (e.g., too much or too little of specific hormones and salts in the blood)
- Malnutrition (e.g., too much or too little food, not enough proteins, vitamins, or minerals)
- Parasites (e.g., bacteria, viruses, amoebas, worms)

Students learning to be doctors or nurses in medical schools throughout the modern world are taught this kind of naturalistic explanation. However, there are actually several different naturalistic medical systems in use today. In Latin America, many people still also rely on humoral pathology to explain and cure their illnesses. This is especially true in rural areas among less educated people.

BODY DEFENCES: IMMUNITY AND IMMUNIZATION

Immunization is a subject that evokes very strong opinions and normally stirs up heated debate as to their efficacy, safety, and reliability. The main questions parents have to answer are whether to immunize or not, and if so, when and with which ones.

It is vital that doctors educate their patients as to the pros and cons, indications and contraindications, and risks and benefits of vaccinations in order that the parents can then make an informed choice for their children. By providing a balanced view of the evidence on immunization, naturopathic physicians and other health care providers can help people make clever decisions regarding their health care, and the health care of their dependents.

In looking at infectious disease, there are several components involved in realizing the incidence of these diseases:

- Sanitation
- Nutrition
- Individual emotional, mental, and physical states
- Societal stressors
- The natural progression of the disease
- Natural immunity

By assessing each individual case by these parametres, one can then provide a framework to the parents from which they can make their educated decision regarding immunization.

There are several other criteria which should be evaluated before a decision is made:

- What is the risk or probability of the child getting the disease?
- What are the health consequences of the natural infection if contracted?
- How safe is the vaccine that is available?

- Is the immunity provided by the vaccine solid and long-lasting?
- Will the vaccine stimulate the appropriate parts of the immune system: is the route of vaccine administration compatible with the route of natural infection?
- What is the child's health history and present health condition?
- Are there alternatives to immunization, and if so, are they safe and effective?

Active prevention involves routine immunization of infants and children against diphtheria, tetanus, pertussis, poliomyelitis (Types 1, 2, 3), measles, mumps, and rubella.

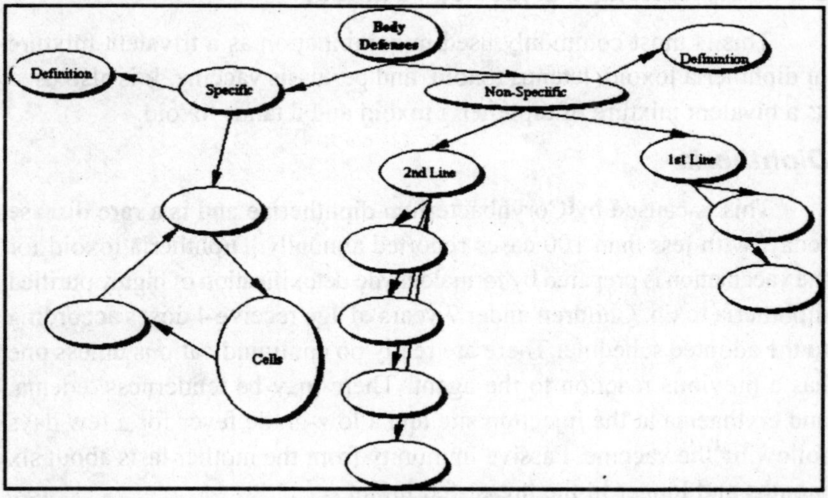

Fig. Body Defences

Any immunizing biologic should be used only in conformity with published recommendations, as their effective use requires reference to the latest rules established by assessment of both past and present knowledge. Some of the risks and contraindications to immunization are:

- Routine immunization should be deferred during acute febrile illness
- Atopic dermatitis or acute skin rash
- Pregnancy
- Hypersensitivity to any vaccine component
- Cases where the patient is undergoing immunotherapy
- Cases where the patient has an altered immunity

The fundamental idea behind immunization is to produce a state of immunity to these childhood infectious diseases through the deliberate, artificial stimulation of the body's defences against each disease. Ideally, this is done without causing any symptoms or signs of illness.

In reality, no immunizing biological agent is completely safe, and it may produce side effects. It is significant to evaluate each person child and each individual vaccine, and then allow the parent to decide what to do after weighing all the facts and sorting out the fiction.

COMMON TYPES OF VACCINATION

DPT (Diphtheria, Pertussis, Tetanus)

This is most commonly used in combination as a trivalent mixture of diphtheria toxoid, tetanus toxoid, and pertussis vaccine. It is also used as a bivalent mixture of diphtheria toxoid and tetanus toxoid.

Diphtheria

This is caused by Corynbacterium diphtheriae and is a rare disease today, with less than 100 cases reported annually. Diphtheria toxoid for the vaccination is prepared by formaldehyde detoxification of highly purified diphtheria toxin. Children under 7 years of age receive 4 doses according to the adopted schedule. There are really no contraindications unless one has a previous reaction to the agent. There may be tenderness, edema, and erythaema at the injection site and a low-grade fever for a few days following the vaccine. Passive immunity from the mother lasts about six months and longer in the breast-fed infant.

Pertussis (Whooping Cough)

This is caused by Bordatella pertussis, with about 2,000 cases reported annually. Pertussis vaccine is a killed whole-cell preparation of a culture of Bordatella pertussis. A series of four doses is given for fundamental immunization, with a booster recommended between ages 4 and 6, according to the adopted schedule. Newborns are susceptible in spite of maternal immunity.

This vaccine is not recommended after age 6 due to the increased risk of side effects. Contradictions include neurological disorders of unfamiliar condition. Side effects include screaming episodes and prolonged, unresponsive crying, fever of 105 or greater, convulsion with or without fever, collapse, encephalopathy, and local inflammatory changes at the site of injection.

Tetanus

Clostridium tetani produces a potent neurotoxin, which, under anaerobic conditions, produces the disease known as lockjaw. There are approximately 100 cases reported annually, with a 40% fatality rate. Immunity to tetanus results from immunizing agents only; the disease does not confer immunity. A newborn infant is immune if the mother is correctly immunized.

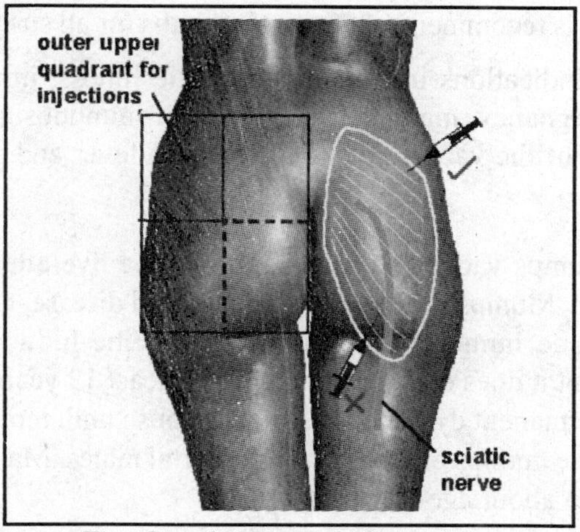

Fig. Site for Tetanus Injection

The tetanus toxoid is a formaldehyde-immunity, with a reinforcing dose every 10 years. The only contraindication is a severe prior reaction to the toxoid. There may be mild inflammation at the site of injection.

Poliomyelitis

There are about 20 cases of polio reported annually. Vaccines used according to the established rules can be protective, with three separate doses given by age 2, and a booster given at about age 5.

Two types of polio vaccine are available:

- Oral polio vaccine (OPV), a live, attenuated virus agent; and
- Inactivated polio vaccine (TOPV), a mixture of all three types of the virus, which is recommended for those under age 18.

Contraindications include immune deficiency diseases, altered immune condition, use of steroids, alkylating agents and antemetabolites, and pregnancy.

MMR (Measles, Mumps, Rubella)

This is often given as a trivalent vaccine at 15 months of age, though each one can be used separately.

Measles

The measles vaccine is a highly attenuated strain of rubella virus. Duration of immunity is not known, though the vaccine is good for at least 15 years. The disease itself, if contracted, offers lifetime immunity. Vaccination is recommended at age 15 months for all susceptible persons.

Contraindications include acute febrile illness, immunodeficiency diseases, pregnancy, malignancy, and use of immunosuppressive drugs. Side effects of the vaccine include moderate fever and skin rash.

Mumps

The mumps vaccine is a preparation of a live attenuated strain of mumps virus. Mumps is normally a self-limited disease, and if contracted, offers lifetime immunity. Duration of vaccine-induced immunity is unknown, but it does offer protection for at least 12 years. Mumps rarely results in permanent dysfunction, but can cause unilateral nerve deafness and can cause mumps orchitis in postpubertal males. Maternal antibodies protect up to about age 12 months.

Mumps vaccine is contraindicated in persons with malignancy, immune deficiency disease, conditions of altered immunity, and in pregnancy. Side effects to the vaccine are normally limited to local mild inflammation at the site of injection.

Nurses working in both community and hospital settings are increasingly undertaking immunization. This may include child immunization regimes, vaccinations for travel abroad, the administration of influenza vaccines and the giving of anti-tetanus or hepatitis B vaccinations within accident and emergency units or treatment rooms.

Jones (1994) examines some of the legal and professional aspects of immunization by nursing staff and discusses the use of protocols for this practice. Nurses participating in any immunization programme must meet the following criteria. They must:

- Undertake additional training on immunization
- Undertake training in the management of anaphylaxis
- Be competent in the practice of immunization and be able to recognise contraindications for vaccination

- Be responsible for their practice.
- Rubella

Rubella infections are prevented by active immunization programs using live, disabled virus vaccines. Two live attenuated virus vaccines, RA 27/3 and Cendehill strains, were effective in the prevention of adult disease. However their use in prepubertile females did not produce a significant fall in the overall incidence rate of CRS in the UK. Reductions were only achieved by immunization of all children.

The vaccine is now given as part of the MMR vaccine. The WHO recommends the first dose is given at 12 to 18 months of age with a second dose at 36 months. Pregnant women are usually tested for immunity to rubella early on. Women found to be susceptible are not vaccinated until after the baby is born because the vaccine contains live virus.

ILLNESS AND ILLNESS BEHAVIOUR

Illness (sometimes referred to as ill-health or ail) can be defined as a state of poor health. It is sometimes considered a synonym for disease. Others maintain that fine distinctions exist. Some have described illness as the subjective perception by a patient of an objectively defined disease.

The mode of being fit includes, as defined by the World Health Organization, a state of complete physical, mental and social well-being and not merely the absence of disease or infirmity". When these conditions are not fulfilled, then one can be considered to have an illness or be ill. Medication and the science of pharmacology are used to cure or reduce symptoms of an illness or medical conditions. Developmental disability is a term used to describe severe, life-long disabilities attributable to mental and/or physical impairments.

PHYSICAL

Conditions of the body or mind that cause pain, dysfunction, or distress to the individual afflicted or those in contact with the individual can be viewed as an illness. Sometimes the term is used broadly to include injuries, disabilities, syndromes, infections, symptoms, deviant behaviours, and atypical variations of structure and function, while in other contexts these may be considered distinguishable categories. A pathogen or infectious agent is a biological agent that causes disease or illness to its host. A passenger virus is a virus that simply hitchhikes in the body of a person or infects the body without causing symptoms, illness or disease.

Foodborne illness or food poisoning is any illness resulting from the consumption of food contaminated with pathogenic bacteria, toxins, viruses, prions or parasites.

MENTAL

Mental illness (or Emotional disability, Cognitive dysfunction) is a broad generic label for a category of illnesses that may include affective or emotional instability, behavioural dysregulation, and/or cognitive dysfunction or impairment. Specific illnesses known as mental illnesses include major depression, generalized anxiety disorder, schizophrenia, and attention deficit hyperactivity disorder, to name a few. Mental illness can be of biological (e.g., anatomical, chemical, or genetic) or psychological (e.g., trauma or conflict) origin. It can impact one's ability to work or go to school and contribute to problems in relationships. Other generic names for mental illness include "mental disorder", "psychiatric disorder", "psychological disorder", "abnormal psychology", "emotional disability", "emotional problems", or "behaviour problem". The term insanity is used technically as a legal term. Brain damage may occur

SOCIAL

Social determinants of health are the social conditions in which people live which determine their health. Illnesses are generally related to social, economic, political, and environmental circumstances. Social determinants of health have been recognized by several health organizations such as the Public Health Agency of Canada and the World Health Organization to greatly influence collective and personal well-being.

TREATMENT

The governmental involvement is vital and may also be needed to study a range of illnesses and treatments. Health care is the prevention, treatment, and management of illness and the conservation of mental and physical well-being through the services offered by the medical, nursing, and allied health professions. The organised provision of such services may constitute a health care system. Before the term "healthcare" became popular, English-speakers referred to medicine or to the health sector and spoke of the treatment and prevention of illness and disease. A patient is any individual who receives medical attention, care, or treatment. The individual is most often ill or injured and is being treated by, or in need of treatment by, a physician or other medical professional. Health consumer or health care consumer is another name for patient, normally used by some governmental agencies, insurance companies, and/or patient groups.

Medical emergencies are injuries or illnesses that pose an immediate threat to a person's health or life which require help from a doctor or hospital. The doctor's specialization of emergency medicine includes techniques for effective handling of medical emergencies and resuscitation of patients. Emergency departments provides initial treatment to patients with a broad spectrum of illnesses and injuries, some of which may be life-threatening and requiring immediate attention.

STUDY OF ILLNESS

Epidemiology is the scientific study of components affecting the health and illness of persons and populations, and serves as the foundation and logic of interventions made in the interest of public health and preventive medicine.

Behavioural medicine is an interdisciplinary field of medicine concerned with the development and integration of psychosocial, behavioural and biomedical knowledge relevant to health and illness. Clinical Global Impression scale to evaluate treatment response in patients with mental disorders. It's "Improvement scale" requires the clinician to rate how much the patient's illness has improved or worsened relative to a baseline state. Mental confusion and decreased alertness may indicate that a chronic illness has gotten worse.

The notion of illness behaviour was largely defined and adopted during the second half of the twentieth century. Broadly speaking, it is any behaviour undertaken by an individual who feels ill to relieve that experience or to better define the meaning of the illness experience. There are many different types of illness behaviour that have been studied. Some persons who experience physical or mental symptoms turn to the medical care system for help; others may turn to self-help strategies; while others may decide to dismiss the symptoms.

In everyday life, illness behaviour may be a mixture of behavioural decisions. For instance, an individual faced with recurring symptoms of joint pain may turn to complementary or alternative medicine for relief. However, sudden, sharp, debilitating symptoms may lead one directly to a hospital emergency room.

In any event, illness behaviour is normally mediated by strong subjective interpretations of the meaning of symptoms. As with any type of human behaviour, many social and psychological components intervene and determine the type of illness behaviour expressed in the individual.

SICK-ROLE BEHAVIOUR

The sick role is a notion arising from the work of the significant American sociologist Talcott Parsons (1902-1979). Parsons was a structural functionalist who argued that social practices should be seen in terms of their function in maintaining order or structure in society. Thus Parsons was concerned with realizing how the sick individual related to the whole social system, and what the person's function is in that system. Ultimately, the sick role and sick-role behaviour could be seen as the logical extension of illness behaviour to complete integration into the medical care system. Parsons' argument is that sick-role behaviour accepts the symptomatology and diagnosis of the established medical care system, and thus allows the individual to take on behaviours compliant with the expectations of the medical system. Fundamentally, Parsons defined the "sick role" as having four chief characteristics. First, the sick individual is freed or exempt from carrying out normal social roles. The more severe the illness, the more one is freed from normal social roles. Everyone in society experiences this; for instance, a minor chest cold "allows" one to be excused from small obligations such as attending a social gathering. By contrast, a major heart attack "allows" significant time away from work and social obligations. Second, people in the sick role are not directly accountable for their plight. Third, the sick individual needs to try to get well. The sick role is regarded as a temporary stage of deviance that should not be prolonged if at all possible. Finally, in the sick role the sick individual or patient must seek competent help and cooperate with medical care to get well. This conceptual schaema implies many reciprocal relations between the sick individual (the patient), and the healer (the physician). Thus the job of the physician is one of social control.

The complicated theoretical explanations of Parsons yielded a voluminous research literature in the second half of the twentieth century, and they continue to stimulate much research today. In particular, there has been much study of the norms and values that define the behaviours of both the sick and those providing treatment. These studies form the basis for present-day research on the patient-physician relationship. They inform the various strategies undertaken by behavioural scientists to intervene in this relationship to bring about positive behavioural changes in both patient and practitioner that will lead to better health outcomes.

CONCEPTS OF ILLNESS BEHAVIOUR AND SICK-ROLE BEHAVIOUR IN PUBLIC HEALTH

In present-day public health practice, which is based on population and community-based approaches with an emphasis on participation, the research from these notions of behaviour has helped immensely in clarifying critical approaches to public health. The notion of diversity in populations has been greatly enhanced through the articulation of the notions of illness behaviour and the sick role. Researchers now have a important body of research showing the wide variation in these behaviours with respect to all the key demographic variables. For instance, there has been excellent work showing how the presentation of symptoms to a physician is highly dependent on gender, ethnic background, and other sociocultural characteristics. Research on the sick-role notion has elucidated the issue of power and its many manifestations in doctors' offices, hospitals, and other medical settings. It would be difficult, given this literature, for a practicing health educator not to consider the role of power in patient-physician interactions.

Present-day health education has also been heavily determined by the research on illness and sick-role behaviour. These notions have helped inform part of the scientific basis for the educational and environmental approach to health promotion planning elucidated by L. W. Green and M. W. Kreuter in their widely used PRECEDE-PROCEED model. At the same time, the conceptual components of illness and sick-role behaviour continue to be explored in narrative analyses of the written and spoken traditions of peoples to describe their experiences of illness and sickness.

IMPACT OF ILLNESS ON PATIENT AND FAMILY

An entirely traditional biomedical perspective cannot embrace the range of psychological and social components involved in a person's course of illness. The patient's active participation in his or her own health care is significant for the process of adaptation to and recovery from illness. Therefore, patient satisfaction with consultations in general practice has gained significance as a measure of health outcome. Patient satisfaction with domains of health care such as availability and accessibility, organization and cooperation, medical care, information and support, and the relation and communication between patient and physician have been identified and studied. Patient satisfaction has been found to be associated with outcomes such as change of health care provider, quality of treatment, and improved health condition and is used for intentions such as assessment of the quality of health care and identification of components to change to improve satisfaction.

Family members, spouses and partners, and friends of patients are obviously impacted by a patient's illness. While these significant persons spend far more time with patients than either physicians or the mental health professionals who provide care, family members are frequently, albeit unintentionally, left out as significant players in the care and management of persons who are chronically ill. There are likely many reasons for this. First, busy physicians may not feel they have the time to devote to family members. Especially for patients that are seriously ill, conversations with family members can be long and involved. Second, some family members may feel intimidated by physicians or see physicians as the ultimate authority. This is especially true among elderly persons or persons from cultures in which authority is given high respect. In such cases, family members may feel uncomfortable with asking a physician questions or taking an active role in the patient's care. Additionally, many family members are aware of the needs of the patient and seem intentionally to keep a low profile when around physicians so as not to interfere with their loved one's care. Third, in some instances, physicians are under intense pressure to provide concrete answers to family members regarding a patient's condition and prognosis. In some cases, often involving very sick patients, physicians cannot provide definite answers regarding the prognosis and avoid having discussions with family members as a result.

HEALTH CARE SERVICES

HEALTH PROMOTION AND PREVENTION

Health promotion is the process of enabling people to increase control over, and to improve, their health. To reach a state of complete physical, mental and social well-being, an individual or group must be able to identify and to realize aspirations, to satisfy needs, and to change or cope with the environment. Health is, hence, seen as a resource for everyday life, not the objective of living. Health is a positive notion emphasizing social and personal resources, as well as physical capacities. Therefore, health promotion is not just the duty of the health sector, but goes beyond fit life-styles to well-being.

Prerequisites for Health

The fundamental conditions and resources for health are:

- Peace,
- Shelter,
- Education,
- Food,
- Income,
- A stable eco-system,

- Sustainable resources,
- Social justice and equity.

Improvement in health requires a secure foundation in these fundamental prerequisites.

Advocate

Good health is a major resource for social, economic and personal development and a significant dimension of quality of life. Political, economic, social, cultural, environmental, behavioural and biological components can all favour health or be harmful to it. Health promotion action aims at making these conditions favourable through advocacy for health.

Enable

Health promotion focuses on achieving equity in health. Health promotion action aims at reducing differences in current health condition and ensuring equal opportunities and resources to enable all people to achieve their fullest health potential. This includes a secure foundation in a supportive environment, access to information, life skills and opportunities for making fit choices. People cannot achieve their fullest health potential unless they are able to take control of those things which determine their health. This must apply evenly to women and men.

Mediate

The prerequisites and prospects for health cannot be ensured by the health sector alone. More significantly, health promotion demands coordinated action by all concerned: by governments, by health and other social and economic sectors, by nongovernmental and voluntary organization, by local authorities, by industry and by the media. People in all walks of life are involved as persons, families and communities. Professional and social groups and health personnel have a major duty to mediate between differing interests in society for the pursuit of health.

Health promotion strategies and programmes should be adapted to the local needs and possibilities of individual countries and regions to take into account differing social, cultural and economic systems.

Health Promotion Actions

Health promotion goes beyond health care. It puts health on the agenda of policy makers in all sectors and at all levels, directing them to be aware of the health consequences of their decisions and to accept their duties for health.

Health promotion policy combines diverse but complementary approaches including legislation, fiscal measures, taxation and organizational change. It is coordinated action that leads to health, income and social policies that foster greater equity. Joint action contributes to ensuring safer and healthier goods and services, healthier public services, and cleaner, more enjoyable environments.

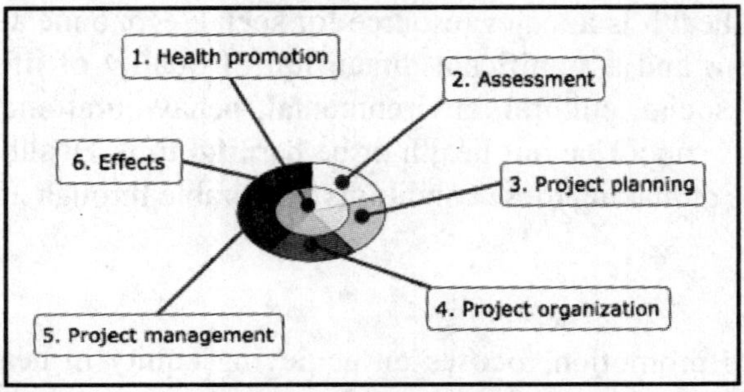

Fig. Health Promotion

Health promotion policy requires the identification of obstacles to the adoption of fit public policies in non-health sectors, and ways of removing them. The aim must be to make the healthier choice the easier choice for policy makers as well.

Creating Supportive Environments

Our societies are complex and interrelated. Health cannot be separated from other goals. The inextricable links between people and their environment constitutes the basis for a socioecological approach to health. The overall guiding principle for the world, nations, regions and communities alike, is the need to encourage reciprocal maintenance - to take care of each other, our communities and our natural environment. The conservation of natural resources throughout the world should be emphasized as a global duty.

Changing patterns of life, work and leisure have a important impact on health. Work and leisure should be a source of health for people. The way society organizes work should help create a fit society. Health promotion generates living and working conditions that are safe, stimulating, satisfying and enjoyable.

Systematic evaluation of the health impact of a rapidly changing environment - particularly in areas of technology, work, energy production and urbanization - is essential and must be followed by action to ensure positive benefit to the health of the public. The protection of the natural and built environments and the conservation of natural resources must be addressed in any health promotion strategy.

Strengthen Community Actions

Health promotion works through concrete and effective community action in setting priorities, making decisions, planning strategies and implementing them to achieve better health. At the heart of this process is the empowerment of communities - their ownership and control of their own endeavours and destinies.

Community development draws on existing human and material resources in the community to develop self-help and social support, and to develop flexible systems for strengthening public participation in and direction of health matters. This requires full and continuous access to information, learning opportunities for health, as well as funding support.

Develop Personal Skills

Health promotion supports personal and social development through providing information, education for health, and enhancing life skills. By so doing, it increases the options available to people to exercise more control over their own health and over their environments, and to make choices conducive to health.

Enabling people to learn, throughout life, to prepare themselves for all of its stages and to cope with chronic illness and injuries is essential. This has to be facilitated in school, home, work and community settings. Action is needed through educational, professional, commercial and voluntary bodies, and within the institutions themselves.

Reorient Health Services

The duty for health promotion in health services is shared among persons, community groups, health professionals, health service institutions and governments. They must work together towards a health care system which contributes to the pursuit of health.

The role of the health sector must move increasingly in a health promotion direction, beyond its duty for providing clinical and curative services. Health services need to embrace an expanded mandate which is sensitive and respects cultural needs. This mandate should support the needs of persons and communities for a healthier life, and open channels between the health sector and broader social, political, economic and physical environmental components.

Reorienting health services also requires stronger attention to health research as well as changes in professional education and training. This must lead to a change of attitude and organization of health services which refocuses on the total needs of the individual as a whole individual.

Moving into the Future

Health is created and lived by people within the settings of their everyday life; where they learn, work, play and love. Health is created by caring for oneself and others, by being able to take decisions and have control over one's life circumstances, and by ensuring that the society one lives in creates conditions that allow the attainment of health by all its members.

Caring, holism and ecology are essential issues in developing strategies for health promotion.

Therefore, those involved should take as a guiding principle that, in each phase of planning, implementation and assessment of health promotion activities, women and men should become equal partners.

Commitment to Health Promotion

The participants in this Conference pledge:

- To move into the arena of fit public policy, and to advocate a clear political commitment to health and equity in all sectors;
- To counteract the pressures towards harmful products, resource depletion, unfit living conditions and environments, and bad nutrition; and to focus attention on public health issues such as pollution, occupational hazards, housing and settlements;
- To respond to the health gap within and between societies, and to tackle the inequities in health developed by the rules and practices of these societies;
- To acknowledge people as the main health resource; to support and enable them to keep themselves, their families and friends fit through financial and other means, and to accept the community as the essential voice in matters of its health, living conditions and well-being;
- To reorient health services and their resources towards the promotion of health; and to share power with other sectors, other disciplines and, most significantly, with people themselves;

- To recognize health and its maintenance as a major social investment and challenge; and to address the overall ecological issue of our ways of living.

Health Promotion Model

The HPM is based on the following assumptions, which reflect both nursing and behavioural science perspectives:

1. Persons seek to create conditions of living through which they can express their unique human health potential.
2. Persons have the capacity for reflective self-awareness, including evaluation of their own competencies.
3. Persons value growth in directions viewed as positive and attempts to achieve a personally acceptable balance between change and stability.
4. Individuals seek to actively regulate their own behaviour.
5. Individuals in all their biopsychosocial complexity interact with the environment, progressively transforming the environment and being transformed over time.
6. Health professionals constitute a part of the interpersonal environment, which exerts influence on persons throughout their lifespan.
7. Self-initiated reconfiguration of person-environment interactive patterns is essential to behaviour change.

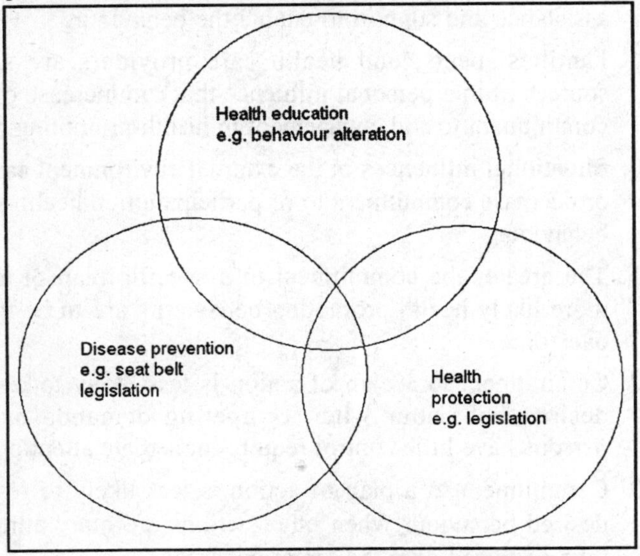

Fig. Health Promotion Model

Theoretical statements derived from the model provide a basis for investigative work on health behaviours. The HPM is based on the following theoretical propositions:

1. Prior behaviour and inherited and acquired characteristics influence beliefs, affect, and enactment of health-promoting behaviour.
2. Persons commit to engaging in behaviours from which they anticipate deriving personally valued benefits.
3. Perceived barriers can constrain commitment to action, a mediator of behaviour as well as actual behaviour.
4. Perceived competence or self-efficacy to execute a given behaviour increases the likelihood of commitment to action and actual performance of the behaviour.
5. Greater perceived self-efficacy results in fewer perceived barriers to specific health behaviour.
6. Positive affect toward a behaviour results in greater perceived self-efficacy, which can in turn, result in increased positive affect.
7. When positive emotions or affect are associated with behaviour, the probability of commitment and action is increased.
8. Persons are more likely to commit to and engage in health-promoting behaviours when important others model the behaviour, expect the behaviour to occur, and provide assistance and support to enable the behaviour.
9. Families, peers, and health care providers are significant sources of interpersonal influence that can increase or decrease commitment to and engagement in health-promoting behaviour.
10. Situational influences in the external environment can increase or decrease commitment to or participation in health-promoting behaviour.
11. The greater the commitment to a specific plan of action, the more likely health-promoting behaviours are to be maintained over time.
12. Commitment to a plan of action is less likely to result in the desired behaviour when competing demands over which persons have little control require immediate attention.
13. Commitment to a plan of action is less likely to result in the desired behaviour when other actions are more attractive and thus preferred over the target behaviour.

14. Persons can modify cognitions, affect, and the interpersonal and physical environment to create incentives for health actions.

PRIMARY CARE

Accident and Emergency Care

- Systems for emergency care.
- Providing Primary Care in the Accident and Emergency Department.
- Recent advances - Accident and emergency medicine.

Caring for Older People

Community services for elderly people - With an ageing population, health problems of the elderly will take centre stage attention and significance in our future health care system. What is the role of primary care doctors in the care of the elderly in such a system? This topic discusses some of the special ageing issues in the development and research on community services for elderly people with mental disorders. These issues, taken together with Normal Aging Index are evenly relevant when considering community services for the elderly population as a whole

Geriatrics, Prevention, and the Remodelling of Medicare Geriatric medicine has focused primarily on the management of acute and chronic diseases in frail older persons, with much less emphasis on the promotion of health and the prevention of disease than there is in health care for children or middle-aged adults. A growing body of knowledge about disease prevention in later life, including significant research by Inouye et al. that is reported in this issue of the Journal, provides a valid basis for strengthening efforts in preventive geriatrics. Given its mission and duty, the Medicare program is well positioned to lead such an effort on a national scale

Roles of Primary Care Nurses

Adult Nurse Practitioner

Adult nurse practitioners provide primary care to adults and provide counselling on health promotion and disease prevention and emphasize wellness. They diagnose and treat acute and chronic health problems. They may work in physicians' offices, primary care clinics, nurse-managed clinics, occupational health clinics or health department clinics to name a few examples.

Family Nurse Practitioner

Family nurse practitioners provide primary health care to patients of all ages. They may work in community health settings, clinics, physician offices, school health, occupational health, home health, and urgent care. They diagnose and treat common health problems, promote wellness and illness prevention, and help patients learn effective self-care. Family nurse practitioners focus on health promotion and disease prevention throughout the life span. They also diagnose and treat acute and chronic health problems.

Geriatric Nurse Practitioner

Geriatric nurse practitioners work with older adults and their families, promoting fit aging, coordinating care, helping manage therapeutic regimens including medications, and maintaining safe independence. They diagnose and treat common health problems of older adults and work collaboratively with elders and their families or important others in managing care. Geriatric nurse practitioners might work in geriatric clinics, parish nursing programs, long term care facilities, or adult day care centres.

Women's Health Nurse Practitioner

These nurse practitioners specialize in primary health care for women. They may work in physicians' offices, community health clinics, or in women's health clinics. They focus on promoting health and preventing illness in women and include prenatal/postpartum care and gynaecology in their clinical practices.

Roles of Advanced Care Nurses

Acute Care Nurse Practitioner Track

Acute care nurse practitioners care for acutely and critically ill adults. As members of a multidisciplinary health care team, they work in intensive care units and hospital units, emergency departments, specialty clinics, and specialty physicians' offices. They focus on evaluation, diagnosis, and management of acute health problems, and provide tertiary restorative and preventive care to patients and their families.

Adult Clinical Nurse Specialist Track

Adult clinical nurse specialists provide advanced clinical care, patient and staff education, collaborate with other health care professionals throughout the system to improve quality of care, serve as consultants for complex health care problems, and design innovative, evidence-based interventions. They may work in hospitals, clinics or managed care settings.

These specialists focus on helping people make transitions from one level of care to another and often work with those who have acute and chronic health problems. Specializations are available in cardiovascular, oncology, critical care, complementary practices, and other areas.

Nursing Management Track

Nurse Managers play a key role in assuring high quality care and a satisfying work environment on individual units, clinics and departments in all types of health care organizations. They plan, design, implement and evaluate evidence-based clinical programs that are client-centred. Nurse Managers develop policies and procedures that ensure patient safety, promote high quality clinical care, and provide a satisfying and meaningful working environment. They select and hire nursing staff and promote professional development of staff nurses. They monitor budgets and ensure fiscally sound nursing practice in their areas and facilitate teamwork and positive interdisciplinary working relationships.

Community-based Nursing

Registered nurses work to promote health, prevent disease and help patients cope with illness. They are advocates and health educators for patients, families and communities. RNs develop and manage nursing care plans, and instruct patients and their families in proper care to improve or maintain their health.

Community-based nurses work in government and private settings and agencies, clinics, schools, retirement communities and other community settings. They work with community leaders, teachers, parents and physicians to improve the overall health of communities and instruct persons, families, and other groups in health education, disease prevention, nutrition and child care.

Community-based nursing is defined as a philosophy of nursing that guides nursing care for persons, families, communities and populations wherever they are encountered. It fosters the development of partnerships with clients and other disciplines, involves direct and indirect nursing care across the health-illness continuum, develops capacity for self care, incorporates an appreciation of client values, and promotes autonomy in decision making. It guides care in all areas of nursing practice.

Professional nursing is defined as the art and science oriented toward health promotion, risk reduction, disease prevention, illness and disease management and death with dignity. The professional nurse partners with clients to assist them toward independence and their optimal level of wellness through the diagnosis and treatment of actual or potential health problems. The professional nurse collaborates with members of the interdisciplinary team in the (client's) adaptive process to optimize health. The role of the nurse includes provider, designer, manager, and coordinator of care; advocate; educator; researcher; and member of a profession. The major processes that support these roles include critical thinking, communication, evaluation, and acquisition and use of technical skills.

Concepts of this framework are as follows:

- Community-based Nursing related to Clients: Community-based nursing guides nursing care for clients wherever encountered and assists them toward their highest level of wellness.
- Clients related to the Environment: Clients live in communities and are determined by conditions in the biological, physical, chemical, psychosocial, cultural, economic, and political milieu.
- Environment related to Health: The dynamic states of health and illness are determined by environmental conditions and by client's and caregivers' responses to the environment.
- Health related to Clients: The state of wellness and illness determines the client's level of capacity for self care and autonomy in decision making.
- Clients related to Professional Nursing: Partnering with clients to assist them toward independence and their optimal level of wellness through the diagnosis and treatment of actual and potential health problems.

Non-relational Propositions Related to the Community-Based Nursing Model

Nursing practice and nursing education may occur when ever and where ever people are encountered in communities.

Community-based nursing requires partnerships with clients and members of other disciplines: to develop effective interventions for persons, families, groups, communities and populations; and to assist them toward independence and optimal levels of health.

These partnerships are ongoing and true partnerships in which: the partners work collaboratively; and the voices of the clients, their families, groups, communities and populations are heard.

Partnering with communities provides nurses with a realistic understanding of the choices and the compromises that occur in the daily lives of the clients; and the impact that the community has on their lives and health.

The interventions that partners develop are: in response to the needs identified by the community; and emerge from the capabilities of the partners.

DIAGNOSIS

By definition, diagnosis is the careful, critical study of something to determine its nature. The question is not whether nurses can diagnose, but what nurses can diagnose.

In 1953, V. Fry introduced the term nursing diagnosis to describe a step necessary in developing a nursing care plan. Over the next 20 years, references to nursing diagnosis appeared sporadically in the literature. From 1973 (the first meeting of the National Group for the Classification of Nursing Diagnosis) to the present, nevertheless, references to nursing diagnosis in the literature have increased tenfold.

Nursing diagnosis is a clinical judgment about individual, family, or community responses to actual or potential health problems/life processes. Nursing diagnosis provides the basis for selection of nursing interventions to achieve outcomes for which the nurse is responsible.

A nursing diagnosis is a standardized statement about to the health of a client (individual, family, or community) for the intention of providing nursing care.

Nursing Diagnosis: Process or Outcome

A review of the literature reveals that, over time, the term nursing diagnosis has been used in three contexts:

1. As the second step of the nursing process. In this step, the nurse analyzes data collected during evaluation and evaluates the client's health condition. Some conclusions resulting from data analysis lead to nursing diagnoses; others do not. It is significant to recognize that the outcome of this process can include problems treated primarily by nurses and problems requiring treatment by professionals from several disciplines. For instance, while evaluating a particular client, the nurse may record observations that point to the medical problems of seizures, pneumonia, and hypertension, as well as the nursing diagnosis of Risk for Injury. Using the term nursing diagnosis to designate the second step of the nursing process may be

confusing and have the undesirable effect of leading nurses to try to state all conclusions or problems as nursing diagnoses.

2. As a list of diagnostic labels or titles. After the first conference on nursing diagnosis in 1973, the term nursing diagnosis was applied to specific labels describing health states that nurses could legally diagnose and treat. These labels are concise descriptors of a cluster of signs and symptoms, such as Anxiety, or of increased vulnerability, such as Risk for Injury.

3. As a two-part or three-part statement. Nurses use the term nursing diagnosis to describe a two-part or three-part statement about an individual's, a family's, or a group's response to a situation or health problem.

   Thus, it has become necessary to indicate clearly whether the term nursing diagnosis is being used in the context of problem identification, a classification system of diagnostic labels, or an individualized diagnosis. To avoid misuse and confusion, the author recommends using the following terms:

- For the second step of the nursing process: diagnosis
- For the list of diagnostic labels or titles: diagnostic label or nursing diagnosis
- For the diagnostic statement: nursing diagnosis

HEALTH CARE TEAMS

ATTENDING PHYSICIANS

An attending doctor (often called the "staff" doctor) leads the health care team and has overall duty for care while the patients are in the hospital. Along with resident doctors, the attending doctor examines you, monitors daily progress, plans care, and oversees treatment.

RESIDENTS

Residents are licensed doctors who are receiving additional specialty training. During their residency program, they provide care under the supervision of the attending doctor. Residents are in the hospital 24-hours a day, seven days a week, and hav• close contact with patients and families.

FELLOWS

Fellows are licensed doctors who have completed a residency program and are completing additional advanced training in another specialty area.

PHYSICIAN ASSISTANTS

Physician assistants are health professionals licensed to practice medicine with doctor supervision. They make medical decisions and provide a broad range of diagnostic and therapeutic services.

NURSES

Many types of nurses will help care for you. They provide care and treatment and will be a very significant part of your daily experience.

REGISTERED NURSES

Registered nurses (R.N.) are accountable for all general nursing care and for teaching patients and their families.

NURSING ASSISTANTS

A nursing assistant (N.A.) will be assigned to you each shift to support the nursing team.

NURSE MANAGERS

Nurse managers (N.M.) are accountable for the overall leadership of the unit and are a resource for patients and families who need help resolving problems or addressing concerns.

ASSISTANT NURSE MANAGERS

Assistant nurse managers (A.N.M.) support nurse managers as required.

ADVANCED REGISTERED NURSE PRACTITIONERS

An advanced registered nurse practitioner (A.R.N.P.) has additional education in a specialty area. These nurses work closely with attending doctors and nursing staff to provide your care.

NURSING UNIT CLERKS

The nursing unit clerks provide clerical support for each unit and communicate patient and family requests to others on the care team. They assist with patient admission, transfer, and discharge. The unit clerk can answer many of your questions about non-medical hospital services.

DIETICIANS

Dieticians help ensure that you receive appropriate nutrition to support healing. They are available to explain special diets if required..

OCCUPATIONAL THERAPISTS

These staff members evaluate your motor, sensory, cognitive, perceptual, and psychosocial development. They help patients gain maximum independence in their daily life.

PHARMACISTS

Pharmacists prepare and dispense medications. They work closely with doctors and nurses to monitor drug therapies and to prevent or correct drug interactions. They are available to answer any questions you may have about your medicines.

PHLEBOTOMISTS

These staff members draw blood for laboratory tests.

PHYSICAL THERAPISTS

Physical therapists evaluate the patient's developmental and functional skills. They treat physical, developmental, and neurological problems, and help you learn to use your body through exercise.

RESPIRATORY THERAPISTS

Respiratory therapists evaluate and treat patients with breathing problems. They provide oxygen and other therapies, monitor ventilator functions, and offer education and equipment to patients who need ongoing respiratory care.

SOCIAL WORKERS

Social workers help families with emotional, physical, and financial concerns related to your illness. They are available to help during treatment, hospitalization, and discharge. Social workers refer families to financial and social service resources and coordinate with community and educational agencies near your home.

STUDENTS

It is possible that students from many health-related fields will be active and helpful in your care. They work closely with our staff and are held to the same standards regarding patient confidentiality and practice as the hospital staff. Students do not make independent decisions about your care.

VOLUNTEERS

Volunteers are significant members of the health care team.

TYPES OF HEALTH CARE AGENCIES

There is a direct connection between nursing actions and the health of the environment in health care agencies. However, in daily practice nurses, whether administering a medication, changing a dressing, or starting an IV, do not normally consider the environmental impact of such activities. For instance, discarding wrappers that represent by-products of their work is an almost subliminal activity in their professional role since their focus as a nurse is more frequently on other priorities.

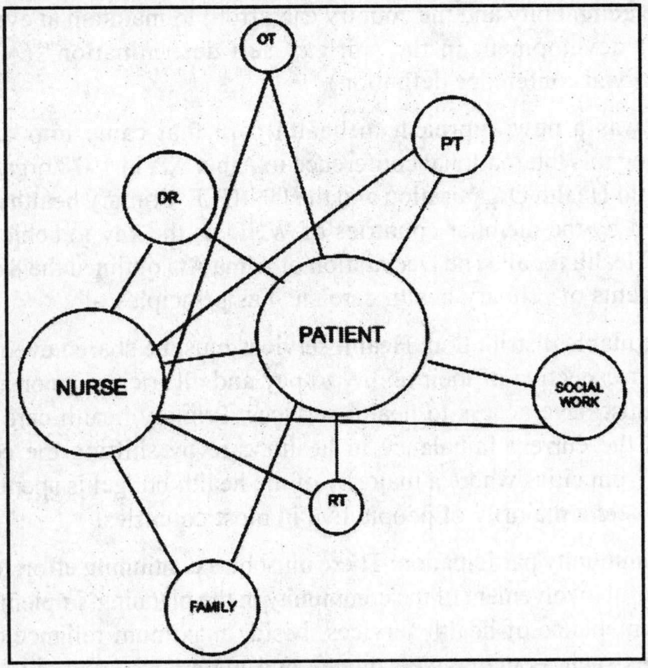

Fig. Health Care Teams

To recognize the unconscious nature of many of nursing activities that do impact the environment, such as waste disposal, nurses need to take a moment and reflect on the last time they worked. It helps to do an evaluation of the many items handled in a given shift that could have a negative effect on the environment. Try this evaluation yourself by replaying (evaluating) the activities of a shift. For instance, consider how many medications were administered, what types of supplies were used, how many units of blood were hung, how many forms were filled out, how many items went from a nurse's hands to a sharps container, a trash can, a recycling bin, a red bag, or a hazardous chemical waste container. Ask yourself how many gallons of water were used to complete toileting and bathing patients? How much electrical energy was used in caring for patients? Then make your diagnoses, i.e., think about the environmental impact of all of these common, daily nursing activities.

PRIMARY HEALTH CARE SERVICES

Primary health care, often abbreviated as PHC, is "essential health care based on practical, scientifically sound and socially acceptable methods and technology made universally accessible to persons and families in the community through their full participation and at a cost that the community and the country can afford to maintain at every stage of their development in the spirit of self-determination" (Alma Ata international conference definition)

It was a new approach to health care that came into existence following this international conference in Alma Ata in 1978 organized by the World Health Organisation and the UNICEF. Primary health care was accepted by the member countries of WHO as the key to achieving the goal of Health for all. The Declaration of Alma Ata outlined the 8 essential components of primary health care such as principles of:

Equitable distribution: Health services must be shared evenly by all people irrespective of their ability to pay and all (rich or poor, urban or rural) must have access to health services. Primary health care aims to address the current imbalance in health care by shifting the centre of gravity from cities where a majority of the health budget is spent to rural areas where a majority of people live in most countries.

Community participation: There must be a continuing effort to secure meaningful involvement of the community in the planning, implementation and maintenance of health services, beside maximum reliance on local resources such as manpower, money and materials.

Intersectoral coordination: Primary health care involves in addition to the health sector, all related sectors and aspects of national and community development, in particular agriculture, animal husbandry, food, industry, education, housing, public works, communication and other sectors.

Four Cornerstones in primary health care are:

1. Active community participation
2. Intra and Inter-sectoral linkages
3. Use of appropriate Technology
4. Support Mechanism made Available

Elements of PHC: Education for health Locally endemic disease control Expanded program of immunization Maternal and child health Essential drugs Nutrition Treatment of communicable disease safe water and sanitation.

SECONDARY HEALTH CARE SERVICES

The term secondary care is a service provided by medical specialists who generally do not have first contact with patients, for instance, cardiologists, urologists and dermatologists. A physician might voluntarily limit his or her practice to secondary care by refusing patients who have not seen a primary care provider first, or a physician may be needed, normally by various payment agreements, to limit the practice this way.

In the United States, nevertheless, there is a trend toward self-referral by patients for these services, rather than referral by primary care providers. This is quite different from practice in the United Kingdom and Canada, for instance, where all patients must first seek care from primary care providers who will in turn decide whether to refer the patient to secondary or tertiary care providers. In Canada, secondary care providers will not be paid by the publicly funded health care system unless the patient has been assessed by a primary care provider (a hospital emergency room doctor is considered a primary care provider, as is a general practitioner or family doctor).

TERTIARY HEALTH CARE SERVICES

In medicine, tertiary healthcare is specialized consultative care, normally on referral from primary or secondary medical care personnel, by specialists working in a centre that has personnel and facilities for special investigation and treatment.

Specialist cancer care, neurosurgery (brain surgery), burns care and plastic surgery are examples of tertiary care services. In comparison, secondary medical care is the medical care provided by a physician who acts as a consultant at the request of the primary physician.

FUNCTIONS AND PURPOSES OF THE HEALTH CARE AGENCIES

A health care provider or health professional is an organization or individual who delivers proper health care in a systematic way professionally to any individual in need of health care services. Health care professionals include physicians, physician assistants, support staff, nurses, pharmacists, therapists, psychologists, veterinarians, dentists, chiropractors, physical therapists, optometrists, paramedics, and a wide variety of other persons regulated and/or licensed to provide some type of health care.

The goals for health systems, according to the World Health Report 2000 - Health systems: improving performance (WHO, 2000), are good health, responsiveness to the expectations of the population, and fair financial contribution. Duckett (2004) proposed a two dimensional approach to assessment of health care systems: quality, efficiency and acceptability on one dimension and equity on another.

HOSPITALS: TYPES, ORGANISATION AND FUNCTIONS

Finding out whether a hospital offers specialized or general care, whether the hospital is a teaching hospital, or whether it is a non-profit or for-profit institution can mean different levels of care and competency. This should be discussed with your doctor so that you can make an informed decision.

TEACHING HOSPITALS

Teaching hospitals are almost always affiliated with a medical school. This can mean access to highly skilled specialists who teach at the school and are the best and brightest in their specialty. It could also mean you will be treated by student doctors with varying levels of experience and talent.

The risk of falling into the hands of such doctor generally increases the busier the hospital and the weaker its financial condition. It is highly advisable that you consult with your physician about the appropriateness of a teaching hospital.

COMMERCIAL HOSPITALS

These are profit-making businesses. Also known as, proprietary hospitals are normally owned by corporations or medical partnerships. Some consumer advocates have argued that these types of business models are more prone to substandard care such as a premature discharge of a patient or the failure to order costly medical testing.

Most people believe these problems are really derived from the managed care dilemma, which can place profit before the best interests of the patient. Hospitals quickly develop reputations among the medical community. Don't be shy to ask your doctor which hospitals are known for quality and compassionate care.

NON-PROFIT AND FOR-PROFIT HOSPITALS

Although the quality of care varies widely within each of these two categories, learning who owns the hospital is key to anticipating the type of care to expect.

NON-PROFIT COMMUNITY HOSPITALS

This type of hospital operates under a religious affiliation or under some other form of voluntary support. Ultimate duty for the care given rests with a board of trustees, who normally are appointed and serve without pay.

THE ROLE AND FUNCTION OF HOSPITALS

A hospital may undertake several functions, depending on the type of hospital, its role in the health care system and its relationship with other health care services. The questions usually asked by policy-makers include: What size population should the hospital serve? How many patients, beds and specialties should it contain? Where should the boundary lie between the hospital and other health services? The answers will depend on the values and objectives of the individual or organization asking the questions. In many cases, competing objectives must be balanced. For instance, surgeons may want large hospitals that can support large clinical teams and complex equipment, whereas the public may want 'their' hospital close to where they live.

Functions of an Acute Care Hospital

The core function of a hospital is to treat patients who are ill, but an analysis confined to this function would be misleading. The hospital may also be an significant setting for teaching and research and may actively support its surrounding health care system. Furthermore, the hospital may be a significant source of local employment and may play several societal roles. The expectations that accompany each of these roles have significant implications for the organization of the hospital and its relationship with its wider environment.

DIFFERENT TYPES OF HOSPITALS

The preceding section explored the roles and functions of the hospital. There are significant differences between types of hospitals. For instance, some hospitals may not engage in teaching or research and, in small communities, the hospital may take on an extended range of social roles. Types of hospitals can be grouped under a hierarchical classification: tertiary care (often a national or regional resource and usually linked with universities), secondary care (such as district hospitals) and community or rural hospitals. An additiónal dimension is added by distinguishing between specialist and general hospitals. The limitation of these simple classifications is becoming clearer, especially the division between secondary and tertiary care hospitals, which is increasingly blurred in high-income countries. For instance, a 'district' hospital in India may have a team of surgeons, each specializing in breast or endocrine surgery, gastrointestinal surgery or vascular surgery, and with specialist support staff. In contrast, in poorer countries, 'general' surgeons may operate on all of these conditions.

TERTIARY CARE HOSPITALS

Tertiary care hospitals are defined, strictly, as those receiving patients referred from secondary care hospitals. Tertiary care hospitals offer the most complex and technologically sophisticated services, are normally linked to a medical school and are generally a regional-level resource. The notion of a tertiary hospital is based on the premise that scarce expertise and expensive equipment need to be concentrated in a few central facilities to which only the patients requiring specialized care are referred. A tertiary care hospital may be 30-day mortality, percentage of hospital-caused (nosocomial) infections, percentage of 'medical mistakes' among patients and emergency readmission within 28 days of discharge either a general hospital (housing many specialties) or a specialist hospital (concentrating on a population group, illness or technique). A general tertiary hospital normally houses specialties such as cardiac surgery, neurosurgery, transplant surgery and advanced cancer treatment.

SPECIALIST HOSPITALS

Specialist hospitals proliferated in the late nineteenth century, reflecting increasing specialization within the medical profession. These hospitals acquired medical and social condition, since they housed the medical elite and were thus regarded as extremely desirable by both staff and patients. Specialist hospitals included maternity, paediatrics, orthopaedic surgery, neurology, ear, nose and throat surgery and ophthalmology. In most western European countries, with a few exceptions, this model gave way to the 'general hospital' from the late 1940s onwards.

DISTRICT GENERAL HOSPITALS

A district general hospital in a high-income country normally serves a population of between 150,000 and 1 million inhabitants. District hospitals treat people for conditions that require more complex treatment than can be provided in a primary care setting or in an ambulatory setting. These hospitals normally have between 200 and 600 beds and normally provide inpatient and outpatient. Many countries have a lower tier of hospital, sometimes called a community hospital. These normally have 50 beds or less and provide fundamental diagnostic services, minor surgery and care for patients who need nursing care but not the facilities of a district general hospital. Small community hospitals exist in some areas because of long distances between scattered communities and the lack of general physicians in remote areas.

THE CHANGING HOSPITAL

Modern acute care hospitals must engage in a continuing process of reconciling several functions: patient care, teaching and research, health system support, employment and wider societal functions. Hospitals in present time are busier places, with more and sicker patients being admitted for shorter lengths of time for more intensive treatment. Patient management within the hospital is also changing, with more patients being treated as day cases. In response, the staffing, design of hospitals and organization of work has to be re-engineered. Old ways of classifying hospitals also no longer apply as new technology becomes more widely available to district and not just strictly tertiary care hospitals.

HEALTH PROMOTION AND LEVELS OF DISEASE PREVENTION

There is a need for solid knowledge with regards to individual, social and wider contextual determinants of relevant health outcomes. Justification for proposed preventive interventions should be grounded in knowledge about the causes of health and disease. In general, causality is fundamental in relation to two fundamental components of evidence-based prevention:

- Demonstrating the causes of a given health problem and
- Furnishing insight into the likelihood and character of causal relations between an intervention and its effect.

This type of evidence predominantly builds on epidemiological studies and approaches. Evidence of the determinants of health and disease provides knowledge of the significance and nature of examined risk components for health at the individual and population levels. Furthermore, it is used to evaluate the preventability of various health problems. To give one example: Epidemiological knowledge shows that physical inactivity leads to lower life expectancy. Sedentary lifestyle is also linked to sizeable losses of health-related quality of life. At the same time we know that physical inactivity is not an unchangeable state. There are effective ways to promote exercise and active living. This type of insight shows that something can and should be done to counteract low levels of physical activity. Typically, the first answer to queries such as these takes off from an analysis of the health condition of specified populations. A classic example is constituted by public surveys of the nature and impact of health-related problems affecting the individual and the wider community.

Epidemiology is the study of the distribution and determinants of health related states or events in specified populations, and the application of this study to the control of health problems. Surveys, similar to SUSY, are also conducted regularly by a number of regional and municipal authorities, NGO's and private companies. Health profiling is one concrete way to describe the state of health at the individual, community or wider societal level. The content of a health profile varies, but it may include information on lifestyles, living conditions, and various dimensions of health and wellbeing. Typical lifestyle components are tobacco, alcohol consumption, diet, use of prescriptive and non-prescriptive drugs, cultural and leisure activities, stress, and exercise. As to living conditions, the focus may be on family and/or kinship relations, the social surroundings, education, profession, occupation, income, general standard of living, physical environments with an impact on health and health behaviours etc. Information on health conditions may include morbidity and mortality rates, functional capacity, self-rated health evaluation and quality of life. Many health profiles also contain information on the resources and use of health services.

LEVELS OF DISEASE PREVENTION

Preventing any disease can be grouped into three levels. The levels are named for the stages of disease they target. The three levels of prevention are primary, secondary, and tertiary.

The Three Levels of Prevention

Primary Prevention

We use primary prevention methods before the individual gets the disease. Primary prevention aims to prevent the disease from occurring. So primary prevention reduces both the incidence and prevalence of a disease. Encouraging people to protect themselves from the sun's ultraviolet rays is an example of primary prevention of skin cancer.

Secondary Prevention

Secondary prevention is used:

- After the disease has occurred, but
- Before the individual notices that anything is wrong.

A doctor checking for suspicious skin growths is an example of secondary prevention of skin cancer. The goal of secondary prevention is to find and treat disease early. In many cases, the disease can be cured.

Tertiary Prevention

Tertiary prevention targets the individual who already has symptoms of the disease

The goals of tertiary prevention are:

- Prevent damage and pain from the disease
- Slow down the disease
- Prevent the disease from causing other problems (These are called "complications.")
- Give better care to people with the disease
- Make people with the disease fit again and able to do what they used to do

Developing better treatments for melanoma is an example of tertiary prevention. Examples include better surgeries, new medicines, etc.

ROLE OF NURSE IN PRIMARY HEALTH CARE AND ITS DELIVERY

The definition for primary care proposed by health professionals alternates between five generic categories. Each category can be interpreted differently. Sometimes these definitions overlap. Sometimes they do not. These categories include:

- Services rendered by primary care practitioners
- A process, such as the entry point into the health care system
- The organisation of care, or the means by which the two goals of a health services system: optimization of health and equity in distributing resources: are balanced
- A set of attributes characterised by accessibility, coordination, continuity, comprehensiveness and accountability

- Patient-oriented, community-based care, with some definitions of primary health care not only including but also requiring the active participation of nurse practitioners and certified nurse midwives

While broad agreement exists that a core group of physicians qualifies as primary care practitioners, disagreement arises on the designation of other physicians who claim to be primary care providers. It is very significant to settle these claims when designing the health care system around primary care, because it must determine who primary care providers are, how they are going to be paid, and what kinds of incentives they will be offered to organise their practices.

The failure to define primary care by its clinical and technical knowledge and the skills and services that are involved creates vagueness around the notion. Without agreement about a common clinical basis for primary care, there will be disagreements about who provides primary care, how they relate to each other, and how they should relate to their patients. Professional consensus on these issues is a critical step toward building the health care system around primary care to ensure its success.

Though many definitions of primary care which is also known as general practice have been proposed, one of the most frequently quoted is the Leeuwenhorst definition from 1974: "The general practitioner is a licensed medical graduate who gives personal, primary and continuing care to persons, families and a practice population irrespective of age, sex and illness. It is the synthesis of these functions which is unique."

REFERENCES

Andrews, H., & Roy, C. (1991). The Roy adaptation model: The definitive statement. East Norwalk, CT: Appleton & Lange.

Boutain, D. (1999). Critical nursing scholarship: Exploring critical social theory with African-American studies. Advances in Nursing Science, 21(4), 37–47.

Levine, M. (1995). The rhetoric of nursing theory. Image: Journal of Nursing Scholarship. 27(1), 14.

Meleis, A., Sawyer, L., I. E., Hilfinger Messias, D., & Schumacker, K. (2000). Experiencing transitions: An emerging middle-range theory. Advances in Nursing Science, 23(1), 12–28.

Neil, J., & Barrell, L. (1998). Transition theory and its relevance to patients with chronic wounds. Rehabilitation Nurse, 23(6), 295–299.

Newman, M. (1986). Health as expanding consciousness. St. Louis: Mosby.

Orem, D. (1991). Nursing concepts of practice (4th ed.). New York: McGraw-Hill.

Nightingale, F. (1859). Notes on nursing: What it is and what it is not. Printed by Harrison and Sons, London, 1946.

2

Nursing Profession

The term profession is applied to those persons who have specialized and technical skill or knowledge which they apply, for a fee, to certain tasks that ordinary and unqualified people cannot ordinarily undertake. The term derives from the Latin: "to swear (an oath)". The oath referred to dictates adherence to ethical standards, which invariably include practitioner/client confidentiality, truthfulness, and the striving to be an expert in one's calling, all three of these being practiced above all for the benefit of the client. There is also a stipulation about upholding the good name of the profession.

The term profession thus refers to an occupation, vocation or high-status career, normally involving prolonged academic training, formal qualifications and membership of a professional or regulatory body. Professions involve the application of specialized knowledge of a subject, field, or science to fee-paying clientele. It is axiomatic that "professional activity involves systematic knowledge and proficiency." Professions are commonly regulated by professional bodies that may set examinations of competence, act as a licensing authority for practitioners, and enforce adherence to an ethical code of practice.

Nursing is a profession focused on assisting persons, families, and communities in attaining, maintaining, and recovering optimal health and functioning. Modern definitions of nursing define it as a science and an art that focuses on promoting quality of life as defined by persons and families, throughout their life experiences from birth to care at the end of life.

DEFINITION

Though nursing practice varies both through its various specialities and countries, these nursing organizations offer the following definitions:

Nursing covers autonomous and collaborative care of persons of all ages, families, groups and communities, sick or well and in all settings. Nursing includes the promotion of health, prevention of illness, and the care of ill, disabled and dying people. Advocacy, promotion of a safe environment, research, participation in shaping health policy and in patient and health systems management, and education are also key nursing roles.

— International Council of Nurses

The use of clinical judgement in the provision of care to enable people to improve, maintain, or recover health, to cope with health problems, and to achieve the best possible quality of life, whatever their disease or disability, until death."

— Royal College of Nursing UK

Nursing is the protection, promotion, and optimization of health and abilities; prevention of illness and injury; alleviation of suffering through the diagnosis and treatment of human responses; and advocacy in health care for persons, families, communities, and populations.

— American Nurses Association

The unique function of the nurse is to assist the individual, sick or well, in the performance of those activities contributing to health or its recovery (or to peaceful death) that he would perform unaided if he had the necessary strength, will or knowledge.

— Virginia Avenel Henderson

PHILOSOPHY OF NURSING

Nursing is an art and a science dedicated to improving the physical and psychological well-being of patients. Nursing, a scientific discipline, requires creativity in its execution. The art of nursing lies in the application of notions and principles of nursing theory to the design of individualized care using the nursing process. The essence of nursing is to provide evidence-based care to our clients in the performance of those activities that contribute to health promotion, resolution of illness, or end-of-life. This is congruent with Nursing's Social Policy Statement that "nursing is the diagnosis and treatment of human responses to actual or potential health problems."

CHARACTERISTICS, NATURE AND SCOPE OF NURSING PRACTICE

Nurses regardless of specialty or work setting, perform fundamental responsibilities that include treating patients, educating patients and the public about various medical conditions, and providing advice and emotional support to patients' family members. Nurses record patients' medical histories and symptoms, help to perform diagnostic tests and analyze results, operate medical machinery, administer treatment and medications, and help with patient follow-up and rehabilitation.

Long-term care nurses provide medical services on a recurring basis to patients with chronic physical or mental disorders. Medical-surgical nurses provide fundamental medical care to a variety of patients in all health settings. Occupational health nurses provide treatment for job-related injuries and illnesses and help employers to detect workplace hazards and implement health and safety standards. Perianaesthesia nurses provide preoperative and postoperative care to patients undergoing anaesthesia during surgery. Perioperative nurses assist surgeons by selecting and handling instruments, controlling bleeding, and suturing incisions. Some of these nurses also can specialize in plastic and reconstructive surgery. Psychiatric nurses treat patients with personality and mood disorders. Radiological nurses provide care to patients undergoing diagnostic radiation procedures such as ultrasounds and magnetic resonance imaging. Rehabilitation nurses care for patients with temporary and permanent disabilities. Transplant nurses care for both transplant recipients and living donors and monitor signs of organ rejection.

Nurses specializing in treatment of a particular organ or body system commonly are employed in specialty physicians' offices or outpatient care facilities, though some are employed in hospital specialty or critical care units. For instance, cardiac and vascular nurses treat patients with coronary heart disease and those who have had heart surgery, providing services such as postoperative rehabilitation. Dermatology nurses treat patients with disorders of the skin, such as skin cancer and psoriasis. Gastroenterology nurses treat patients with digestive and intestinal disorders, including ulcers, acid reflux disease, and abdominal bleeding. Some nurses in this field also specialize in endoscopic procedures, which look inside the gastrointestinal tract using a tube equipped with a light and a camera that can capture images of diseased tissue.

Some nurses have jobs that require little or no direct patient contact. Most of these positions still require an active Nurse license. Case managers ensure that all of the medical needs of patients with severe injuries and illnesses are met, including the type, location, and duration of treatment. Forensics nurses combine nursing with law enforcement by treating and investigating victims of sexual assault, child abuse, or accidental death. Infection control nurses identify, track, and control infectious outbreaks in health care facilities; develop methods of outbreak prevention and biological terrorism responses; and staff immunization clinics. Legal nurse consultants assist lawyers in medical cases by interviewing patients and witnesses, organizing medical records, determining damages and costs, locating evidence, and educating lawyers about medical issues. Nurse administrators supervise nursing staff, establish work schedules and budgets, and maintain medical supply inventories. Nurse educators teach student nurses and also provide continuing education for Nurses. Nurse informaticists collect, store, and analyze nursing data in order to improve efficiency, reduce risk, and improve patient care. RNs also may work as health care consultants, public policy advisors, pharmaceutical and medical supply researchers and salespersons, and medical writers and editors.

CATEGORIES OF NURSING PERSONNEL

Nurses generally fall into several main groups, depending on where they work: in hospitals, in private practice, in private homes, etc.

HOSPITAL NURSES

Hospital nurses, the largest group, are staff nurses who provide bedside nursing care and carry out the medical regimen prescribed by physicians. They also supervise licensed practical nurses and aides. Hospital nurses are normally assigned to one area such as surgery, maternity, paediatrics, emergency, ICU, or oncology, but they sometimes rotate among departments.

OFFICE NURSES

Office nurses care for outpatients in physicians' offices, clinics, and emergency medical centres. They assist with examinations, administer injections and medications, dress wounds and incisions, assist with minor surgery, and maintain records. Some also perform routine laboratory and office work.

NURSING HOME NURSES

Nurses who work in nursing homes manage care for residents with conditions ranging from a fracture to Alzheimer's disease. Though they often spend much of their time on administrative and supervisory tasks, nursing home nurses also evaluate residents' health, develop treatment plans, supervise licensed practical nurses and nursing aides, and perform invasive procedures, such as starting intravenous fluids. They also work in specialty-care departments, such as long-term rehabilitation units for patients with strokes and head injuries.

PUBLIC HEALTH NURSES

Public health nurses work in government and private agencies, including clinics, schools, retirement communities, and other community settings. They focus on populations, working with persons, groups, and families to improve the overall health of communities.

Public Health Nurses work with communities to help plan and implement programs for immunizations, blood pressure testing, and other health screening. They instruct persons, families, and other groups regarding health issues such as preventive care, nutrition, and childcare.

NURSE PRACTITIONERS

Nurse practitioners are the most advanced nurses, with the power to write prescriptions and independently diagnose and treat patients.

REGISTERED NURSES (RNS)

Registered nurses (RNs) work to promote health, prevent disease, and help patients cope with illness. They are advocates and health educators for patients, families, and communities. When providing direct patient care, they observe, assess, and record symptoms, reactions, and progress in patients; assist physicians during surgeries, treatments, and examinations; administer medications; and assist in convalescence and rehabilitation.

RNs also develop and manage nursing care plans, instruct patients and their families in proper care, and help persons and groups take steps to improve or maintain their health. While State laws govern the tasks that RNs may perform, it is commonly the work setting that determines their daily job responsibilities.

HOME HEALTH NURSES

Home health nurses provide nursing services to patients at home. They evaluate patients' home environments and instruct patients and their families. Home health nurses care for a broad range of patients, such as those recovering from illnesses and accidents, cancer, and childbirth. They must be able to work independently and may supervise home health aides.

Home health nurses provide periodic services, prescribed by a physician, to patients at home. They also provide support to patients and their families, and at times work independently.

OCCUPATIONAL HEALTH NURSES (INDUSTRIAL NURSES)

Occupational health nurses, also called industrial nurses, provide nursing care at worksites to employees, customers, and others with injuries and illnesses. They give emergency care, prepare accident reports, and arrange for further care if necessary. They also offer health counselling, conduct health examinations and inoculations, and evaluate work environments to identify potential or actual health problems.

HEAD NURSES OR NURSE SUPERVISORS

Head nurses or nurse supervisors direct nursing activities, primarily in hospitals. They plan work schedules and assign responsibilities to nurses and aides, provide or arrange for training, and visit patients to observe nurses and to ensure that the patients receive proper care. They also may ensure that records are maintained and equipment and supplies are ordered.

NURSING AS A PROFESSION

The authority for the practice of nursing is based upon a social contract that delineates professional rights and duties as well as mechanisms for public accountability. In almost all countries, nursing practice is defined and governed by law, and entrance to the profession is regulated at national or state level.

The aim of the nursing community worldwide is for its professionals to ensure quality care for all, while maintaining their credentials, code of ethics, standards, and competencies, and continuing their education. There are a number of educational paths to becoming a professional nurse, which vary greatly worldwide, but all involve extensive study of nursing theory and practice and training in clinical skills.

Nurses care for persons who are fit and ill, of all ages and cultural backgrounds, and who have physical, emotional, psychological, intellectual, social, and spiritual needs. The profession combines physical science, social science, nursing theory, and technology in caring for those persons.

In order to work in the nursing profession, all nurses hold one or more credentials depending on their scope of practice and education. A Licensed practical nurse(LPN) works under a Registered nurse. A Registered nurse (RN) provides scientific, psychological, and technological knowledge in the care of patients and families in many health care settings. Registered nurses may also earn additional credentials or degrees enabling them to work under different titles such as:

Clinical Nurse Specialist (CNS), Nurse Practitioner (NP), and Certified Nurse Midwife (CNM)

Nurse Educator - Utilizes educational methodologies to present current information in patient care settings, universities, and communities. Types of nurse educators include: Clinical Instructor, College/University Professor, Staff Development Specialist, and Patient Education Specialist

Nurse Administrator - Coordinates the use of human, financial, and technological resources to provide patient care.

Nurse Researcher - Utilizes statistical methodologies to discover or establish facts, principles or relationships.

There is no profession which offers as many chances for diversified roles as does nursing. Nurses may follow their personal and professional interests by working with any group of people, in any setting, at any time. Some nurses follow the traditional role of working in a hospital setting. Within the hospital setting, nurses may work in areas including:

Critical Care; Emergency; Maternal/Child Care; Medical: Cardiology, Diabetes, Gastroenterology, Gerontology, Nephrology, Neurology, Oncology, Pulmonary, Rehabilitation, Renal, Rheumatology, Urology; Operating Room/Recovery Room; Paediatrics; Psychiatric/Mental Health; Surgical: Burn, Cardiovascular, Ear/Nose/Throat, Gastroenterology, Orthopaedics, Plastic Reconstructive, Transplant

Others may work in non-hospital settings including:

Public/Community Health; Mental Health Agencies; Home Health Care; Physician's Office; Health Maintenance Organizations and Managed Care Companies; Insurance; Occupational Health; Research Centres; Extended Care Facilities; Clinics; Outpatient Surgery Centres; Hospices; Community Schools, Day Care Centres; Military Branches; Independent Practice; Schools of Nursing; Senior Centres, Shelters, Churches

HISTORY OF NURSING IN INDIA

When stating about nursing as a profession, one always gets the picture of Florence Nightingale, the pioneer of nursing profession. She was born to English parents on May 12, 1820 in Florence, Italy. She was titled ' Lady of the lamp'. Her work is well known and well recognized world wide.

She had got the opportunity of good (best) education and also travelled throughout Europe and could make good contacts which really helped her to achieve the "mission" in her life. She came across individuals who were concerned with the reforms of social institutions such as prisons and hospitals. In 1853, she spent three months in Kaiserworth, Germany. In the same year she was appointed as Superintendent of Institution for the care of sick - gentle women in London.

In 1854, during the Crimean war, when women nurses were considered to be revolutionary, Florence Nightingale demonstrated quality nursing care along with 38 other nurses. After her extensive service at the Crimean war, efforts of Florence resulted in the appointment of the Royal Commission on the health of the Army. As one of the consequence, The Army Medical School was founded in 1857.

During her lifetime, her work and devotion enlightened the whole society. She was the founder of Nightingale School for nurses, the first ever of its kind. In 1907, she was conferred "The Order of Merit" by the King.

In 1857 the India Mutiny turned nursing interest to the health of the Army in India. It was for this intention the Royal Commission was appointed in 1859. In 1868, a sanitary department was established.

In March 1888, ten qualified British nurses arrived in India to look after the British Army in India. In 1905, during the British rule in India, missionary nurses arrived as members of Missionary Medical Association. This was the very start of formalized nursing service in India.

Gradually, the increasing need of adequately trained nurses led to creation of South India Examining Board in 1911 and the North India Examining Board in 1912. It was the mission hospital Nursing leaders who laid the foundation of systematic Nursing education in India. However, the mid India Board of Examination was initiated in 1934. But this was not regulated for registration. State-wise councils initiated developing from 1935 onwards. Indian Nursing Council (INC) Act was passed by the Parliament in 1947. The Nursing Council upgraded the educational requirements which permitted only matriculated candidates to seek admission to the schools. Now, India has State-wise registration councils in 19 states.

The Central Government granted an approval to the Bhore Committee's (1946) recommendations by starting two colleges of Nursing in Delhi (1946) and Vellore (1947). This provided university degree level courses. With the efforts of Professor S. Radhakrishnan (the then Chairman of University Education Commission), Nursing education in the country was integrated into the system of higher education.

Over decades, there has been an improvement in the availability of nursing education in India.

NURSING ETHICS

Nursing ethics is a branch of applied ethics that concerns itself with activities in the field of nursing. Nursing ethics shares many principles with medical ethics, such as beneficence, non-malfeasance and respect for autonomy. It can be distinguished by its emphasis on maintaining dignity and collaborative care.

HUMAN RIGHTS AND NURSING PRACTICE

Ethics has been an integral part of nursing practice from the earliest foundations of modern nursing in the late nineteenth century. This has always entailed a respect for human rights of the persons in their care. However, early attempts to define ethics in nursing were focused more on the virtues of the nurses themselves, rather than looking at how the rights of the patient or client might be promoted in particular. In the modern era, the ethics of nursing has shifted more toward the promotion of these rights and the responsibilities of the nurse.

The significance of human rights in nursing was made explicit in a statement adopted by the International Council of Nurses in 1983.

DISTINCTIVE NATURE

Though much of nursing ethics has been derived from medical ethics, there are some components that, arguably, differentiate it. This can be seen by examining beneficence. This is a well established principle of medical ethics, which though acknowledged in nursing ethics, is not applied in the same way. The key difference is that beneficence, when expressed through paternalism, is not considered compatible with nursing ethics. This is because nursing theory seeks a collaborative relationship with the individual in their care. It hence emphasizes respect for the autonomy and dignity of the individual being nursed by promoting choice, rather than paternalistic practice where the health professional chooses what is in the best interests of the individual. Codes of conduct for nurses tend to be written in the ethical framework of deontology and are hence based on the rights of the patient and the responsibilities of the nurse rather than on utilitarian concerns of the consequences justifying the action.

COMMON ETHICAL ISSUES CURRENTLY FACING NURSES

Nursing has traditionally had a subservient role: physicians prescribe and order, nurses carry out the orders. This role is increasingly unsatisfactory to medicine and nursing alike. Better models are emerging but are not yet clearly defined. Nurses began to consider professional independence in the 1960s when nursing research first began to make an impact.

This led to the realization that autonomy meant also greater accountability, and hence professional and legal duty for care given. The production of codes of professional conduct, the necessity of nurses to adhere to them and the revolution in nurse education have sharpened the debate about autonomy. They see university education of nurses and increased capabilities by nurses as decisive components in modifying and expanding the scope of nursing practice. Nursing cannot and does not strive to be independent of other professions, but seeks to be a body with its own skills and areas of expertise, and with a clear understanding of its duties. Concentrating on matters of internal regulation and organization seems to have distracted nursing from pursuing a vision or direction.

As professionals, nurses are responsible for protecting the rights and interests of the client. Consequently, sound nursing practice involves making ethical decision. As professionals, nurses are responsible for protecting the rights and interests of the client. Ethics affects nurses in every health care setting, and each practice setting presents the nurse with its ownset of ethical concerns. For instance, consider home health nursing. With the increased acuity level of clients cared for in the home setting, home health nurses face ever-increasing ethical challenges of continuing to provide quality care under federally mandated cost containment initiatives. Whatever the setting, nurses need to balance their ethical duties to each client with their professional obligations. Often there is an inherent conflict.

ADVOCACY ROLE OF THE NURSE

Patient advocacy refers to speaking on a patient's behalf in order to protect their rights and help them obtain required information and services. The role of patient advocate is frequently assumed by nurses, social workers, and other healthcare providers. Some hospitals, health insurance companies, and other healthcare organizations employ people specifically to assume this role.

A Patient Advocate acts as a liaison between patient and healthcare provider. The Patient Advocate is a vital instrument to both patient and physician in the optimal delivery of healthcare. The advocate is generally knowledgeable in healthcare practices and compliance. The advocate may be present for healthcare appointments and notify the healthcare provider of patient compliance issues and potential physician communication improvements.

Another common theme is confidentiality and is a significant principle in many nursing ethical codes. This is where information about the individual is only shared with others after permission of the person, unless it is felt that the information must be shared to comply with a higher duty such as preserving life.

Also related to information giving is the debate about truth telling in interactions with the individual in care. There is a balance between people having the information needed to make an autonomous decision and, on the other hand, not being unnecessarily distressed by the truth. Generally the balance is in favour of truth telling due to respect for autonomy, but sometimes people will ask not to be told, or may lack the capacity to understand the implications.

REFERENCES

Acton G., Irvin, B., Jensen, B., & Miller, E. (1997). Explicating middle-range theory through methodological diversity. Advances in Nursing Science, 19(3), 78–85.

Barnum, B. (1994). Nursing theory: Analysis, application, evaluation. Philadelphia: Lippincott.

Chinn, P., & Kramer, M. (1995). Theory and nursing: A systematic approach. St. Louis: Mosby.

Eakes, G., Burke, M., & Hainsworth, M. (1998). Middlerange theory of chronic sorrow. Image, 30(2), 179–184.

Fawcett, J. (1984). The metaparadigm of nursing: Present status and future refinements. Image, 16(3), 84–87.

Henderson, V. (1966). The Nature of nursing: A definition and its implication for practice, research, and education. New York: Macmillan.

Kulig, J. (2000). Community resiliency: The potential for community health nursing theory development. Public Health Nurse, 17(5), 374–385.

Leddy, S., & Pepper, J. M. (1993). Conceptual bases of professional nursing (3rd ed.). Philadelphia: Lippincott.

Parse, R. (1987). Nursing science: Major paradigms, theories, and critiques. Philadelphia: Saunders.

Polk, L. (1997). Toward a middle-range theory of resilience. Advances in Nursing Science, 19(3), 1–13.

Rogers, M. (1970). An introduction to the theoretical basis of nursing. Philadelphia: F. A. Davis.

Watson, J. (1989). Watson's philosophy and theory of human caring in nursing. In J. Riehl-Sisca (Ed.), Conceptual models for nursing practice (3rd ed.). Stamford, CT: Appleton & Lange.

3

Admission and Discharge Procees in Hospital

The majority of hospital admissions come through the Emergency Department, which can be considered the primary entrance into a hospital. The remainder of patients are admitted through the doctor's office, either for elective surgery or in preparation for childbirth.

A physician is the only health professional who has the authority to admit and/or discharge patients from a hospital. However, it is significant to understand that physicians do not automatically have the ability to admit patients to any hospital of their choice, but rather, to those where they have "admitting privileges". Physicians must undergo a process to obtain these privileges. Once this process is completed, the physician is "granted privileges" to admit patients to a particular hospital.

It is at the hospital's discretion to approve this process and/or limit which privileges they allow the physician. Furthermore, if a physician transfers his/her patient to another hospital, admission must be arranged through a physician who has admitting privileges at that particular hospital. Once a physician admits a patient to a hospital, the hospital will have its own policies for admitting patients. At the Admitting Department, the patient will be needed to provide personal information, as well as, sign certain consent forms before being taken to the hospital unit. If the individual is critically ill, then, this information is obtained from a family member. The types of illnesses and injuries that require hospitalization are left at the discretion of the admitting physician.

Generally speaking, they include:

- An acute illness that can't be managed at home;
- An illness requiring specialized equipment/treatment processes available only at a hospital;

- An illness that requires acute nursing care and/or monitoring;
- Any condition that requires surgery (e.g., broken bones).

Assessment at a hospital Emergency Department generally involves the following steps:

1. A Triage nurse prioritizes patients for medical evaluation.
2. The Emergency Department physician sees the patient. Depending on the evaluation, the physician may arrange for further evaluation by another health professional such as a specialist, physiotherapist, social worker, etc.
3. The physician determines if admission is needed and, if this is the case, admission is arranged.
4. The physician may determine that the patient is stable enough to go home with follow-up instructions.

ADMISSION TO THE HOSPITAL

Hospital admission involves staying at a hospital for at least one night or more.

PURPOSE

Staying in the hospital overnight is done because the individual is too sick to stay at home, requires 24-hour nursing care, and/or is receiving medications and undergoing tests and/or surgery that can only be performed in the hospital setting.

DESCRIPTION

An individual may be admitted to the hospital for a positive experience, such as having a baby, or because they are undergoing an elective surgery or procedure, or because they are being admitted through the emergency department. Being admitted through the emergency department is the most stressful of these circumstances because the event is unexpected and may be a major life crisis.

Before the individual is taken to their room, admitting procedures are performed. The person's personal data is recorded and entered into the hospital's computer system. This data may include:

- Name
- Address
- Home and work telephone number
- Date of birth

- Place of employment
- Occupation
- Emergency contact information, or the names and telephone numbers of those persons the hospital should contact if the individual being admitted needs emergency care or their condition worsens significantly
- Insurance coverage
- Reason for hospitalization
- Allergies to medications or foods
- Religious preference, including whether or not one wishes a clergy member to visit

PREPARATION

If the hospitalization is prearranged, there are preparations that will make the process go more smoothly. It is helpful to have a list of all medications currently being taken, the dosages, how often they are taken, and the reason for taking them. The list should also include any allergies to food and medications, including a description of the reaction, and when the food or medication was last taken. The list should include over-the-counter (OTC) and prescription medications, vitamins, supplements, and herbal and home remedies.

If the hospital stay involves surgery in which there is the potential for significant blood loss, it may be possible to arrange to have blood drawn and stored so that in the event of a transfusion, the individual receives his or her own blood.

If the hospital stay is an extended one, a list of family and friends, with their telephone numbers, can make it easier to stay in touch with people who can come and visit, or offer support by telephone. It is not a good idea to bring anything of value to the hospital as there are many times when one could be out of the room. However, it may be helpful to have some pocket change available if one needs to make some small purchases at the hospital gift shop, such as a newspaper. If one is going to visit someone in the hospital, change or one dollar bills to use at vending machines may come in handy.

A small bag can be brought into the hospital that contains:

- Night clothes (The hospital supplies their own, but some people like to wear familiar clothing; some people use the hospital outfits to decrease the chance of staining their own clothing or bringing germs home from the hospital.)

- A robe
- Slippers
- Clothes for the return trip home
- Reading material for the hospital stay
- Reading glasses
- Personal care items such as comb, brush, and toothbrush (most hospitals supply these items, but many persons prefer to have their own from home)

It is best not to bring in any medication from home unless it has been prearranged with the physician and hospital staff prior to hospitalization. This is to prevent a mistake from occurring by having the individual taking one dose from their own medicine and then being given another dose from the hospital pharmacy.

ADMISSION PROCEDURE

Pre-admission evaluations are conducted for patients who have planned admissions to hospital. Such evaluations are commonly needed for patients requiring elective procedures. Procedures may include elective surgery, non-invasive tests and medical management. Examples of the latter may include chaemotherapy, dialysis, diabetes stabilisation and obstetrics care. The pre-admission evaluation determines the patient's fitness for procedures and ensures that adequate arrangements are made in preparation for hospitalisation.

For the intentions of the rules, pre-admission evaluation applies only to planned admissions, including both day-only and day-of surgery/ procedure-admissions. Though some patients who are admitted as emergencies also receive pre-admission evaluation, they are not referred to in these rules. Pre-admission processes need to be adapted to suit the individual Health Service requirements.

The rules provide a flexible framework for pre-admission which enables models of care to be responsive to local needs and to changes in health service delivery. Patients have always been assessed prior to procedures, though this previously commenced after the patient had been admitted to hospital. It is now recognised that the pre-admission process can be undertaken prior to the hospital admission. The intention of a pre-admission visit prior to hospitalisation is:

- To optimise the patient's health, ensuring the best medical outcome from the admission by:
- Conducting an anaesthetic evaluation where relevant (this may be performed in an anaesthetic clinic)
- Commencing any necessary pre-admission medication or treatment
- To explain the procedure, risks and expected outcomes to the patient and carer. Options and preferences for hospital care and treatment, as well as patient concerns are discussed
- To obtain the patient's informed consent
- To enable an evaluation concerning:
- Rehabilitation, the presence of a carer, the home environment for convalescence and/ or the requirements for home modifications
- Social issues which need to be attended to (such as financial arrangements, sickness benefits, compensation requirement)
- The delivery of community services if needed.

To assist Health Service plan and implement pre-admission services and processes, common elements of identified best practice have been drawn from existing hospital practice and studies.

- Pre-admission evaluation is conducted on an outpatient basis wherever possible.
- Pre-admission evaluation aims to optimise a patient's health status prior to admission.
- Patients and their carers are the primary focus of pre-admission. They are informed, educated and supported throughout the process.
- Where other health professionals across the continuum of care provide care relating to the condition for which hospital admission is occurring, those practitioners are involved in the pre-admission process.
- Patient information is made available to all relevant providers in an efficient and timely manner.
- Processes for both admission and discharge planning commence during pre-admission.
- Accountability processes are in place to evaluate and improve the pre-admission process.

ROLES AND RESPONSIBILITIES OF NURSES

Nurses are a significant human resource, vital for the delivery of health services in countries across the globe. Recognition of the contribution that the general practice nurse has played in the delivery of primary care can help to develop appropriate delivery and governance structures. A core function of the role is the delivery of care appropriate to need, improving the health and well-being of patients.

Individuals are recognised as best placed to manage their own health needs through the promotion of self care, lifestyle changes and the development of effective strategies to manage their own health needs. Building on the long-term relationships that nurses establish with the population, the nurse's role is fundamental in providing information and support in order to enable patients to make appropriate choices for their health.

SERVICE PROVISION FROM GPNS

Nursing within general practice cannot, and should not, be seen in isolation from other nurses but viewed as part of the whole system of care delivery. The development of key relationships with other nurses and clinicians working in primary and secondary care facilitates the delivery of patient-centred care. As a generalist, the GPN provides nursing services to a broad range of the population, often managing undifferentiated patient needs.

Key services include:

- First-contact evaluation
- Management of long-term conditions
- Promotion of choice and positive health.

Delivery of these services requires skilled, knowledgeable nurses who are responsive to patients' needs and expectations. This requires a flexible approach that makes appropriate use of skills and the significance of ensuring that the practice has enough nursing hours to provide the services that are required. The general practice setting provides an increasing range of roles for both qualified and unqualified nurses.

All roles in general practice nursing should:

- Deliver high-quality, appropriate care in a safe and effective manner
- Listen and hear the patient's needs, and deliver care within this context

- Provide knowledge and support for patients, encouraging them to self manage
- Signpost and refer patients to other clinicians and services
- Be responsible and accountable for patients' care delivery.

Effective skill-mix, including the development and implementation of new roles, is fundamental to delivering responsive services.

These new roles can be confusing for patients, particularly as there is a wide variation of titles used. However, they can be broadly categorised as:

- Assistant practitioners
- General practice nurses
- Senior general practice nurses
- Lead practice nurses
- Advanced practitioners.

Each of these roles should have clear functions, though the generalist nature of general practice does require some overlap, particularly at the margins of each role. Since the impact of increased diagnosis and effective management of long-term conditions will increase the demand for nurse consultations, the mode of care delivery will need to change. This change will include the development of closer working relationships with other organisations, for instance leisure services. To support this, all nurses need to be valued for their own contribution and helped to realise their potential within a structured career pathway.

Not all general practices will require a different nurse working at each level. Thorough analysis of population needs against role definitions will determine the actual skill-mix needed.

A GPN service includes:

- Services delivered to patients
- Nursing contribution to the practice organisation.

SERVICES DELIVERED TO PATIENTS

Patients can expect competent care delivery from nurses working within the GPN service to deliver the services.

Health Promotion

- Opportunistic and planned health promotion and education
- Supporting patients to self care

- Health screening
- Specialist advice (e.g., family planning)
- Women's health services (including cervical cytology and breast awareness)
- Men's health services
- Lifestyle advice, including smoking cessation, exercise and diet
- Vaccination and immunization
- Travel health services

Management of Long-term Conditions

- Identification, diagnosis, monitoring and management of patients with long-term conditions, including diabetes, chronic obstructive pulmonary disease, cardiovascular disease, hypertension, asthma, epilepsy and chronic kidney disease
- Review of medication and adherence to treatments
- Work within practice rules to monitor and advise patients on long-term conditions such as thyroid disorders, rheumatoid arthritis, iron-deficiency anaemia and pernicious anaemia
- Support for patients with mental health problems
- Undertake diagnostic tests and give preventative advice for high-risk patients
- Prescribe medication after completion of a recognised extended nurse-prescribing programme

DISCHARGE FROM THE HOSPITAL

Discharge from the hospital is the point at which the patient leaves the hospital and either returns home or is transferred to another facility such as one for rehabilitation or to a nursing home. Discharge involves the medical instructions that the patient will need to fully recover. Discharge planning is a service that considers the patient's needs after the hospital stay, and may involve several different services such as visiting nursing care, physical therapy, and home blood drawing.

Hospitalization is often a short-term event, so planning for discharge may begin shortly after admission. The physicians, nurses, and case managers involved in a patient's care are part of an evaluation team that keeps in mind the patient's pre-admission level of functioning, and whether the patient will be able to return home following the current hospital admission. Information that could affect the discharge plan should be noted in the patient's medical record so that it will be taken into account when discharge is being scheduled. The primary questions include:

- Can this patient return to his or her preadmission situation?
- Has there been a change in the patient's ability to care for him- or herself?
- Is the patient in need of services to be able to care for him- or herself?
- Which services will the patient need?
- Are there mental health needs that must be met?
- Does the patient agree with the discharge plan?

While an individual has been in the hospital, physicians other than the primary care physician have been in charge of the patient's care. Good discharge planning involves clear communication between the hospital physician(s) and the primary care physician. This may be done by telephone and/or in writing. The information to be conveyed includes:

- A summary of the hospital stay
- A list of test and surgeries performed, with results
- A list of test results still pending
- A list of tests required after discharge, such as a repeat chest x ray
- A list of medications the patient is being discharged with, including the dosage and frequency
- A copy of the patient's discharge instructions
- When the patient should see the primary care physician for a follow-up appointment
- The plan for outpatient treatment, such as home intravenous antibiotics or parenteral nutrition to ensure that duty for this treatment has been clearly transferred and that the primary care physician accepts the treatment duty
- Discharge instructions to the patient on activity level, diet, and wound care

Before leaving the hospital, the patient will receive discharge instructions that should include:

- An explanation of the care the patient received in the hospital

- A list of medications the patient will be taking (the dosage, times, and frequency)
- A list of potential side effects of any newly prescribed medications
- A prescription for any newly prescribed medications
- when to see the primary care physician for a follow-up appointment
- Home Care instructions such as activity level, diet, restrictions on bathing, wound care, as well as when the patient can return to work or school, or resume driving
- Signs of infection or worsening condition, such as pain, fever, bleeding, difficulty breathing, or vomiting
- An explanation of any services the patient will now be receiving, such as for a visiting nurse, and to include contact information

The term discharge planning may be used to refer to the service provided to help patients arrange for services such as rehabilitation, physical therapy, occupational therapy, visiting nurses, or nursing home care. This service may be provided by a case manager or by the hospital's social service department. The patient may request this service, or the physician may make the request in the form of a referral to the department. The patient will need to be evaluated to see what services he or she requires, as well as what services he or she qualifies for (such as meals-on-wheels), or what services the patient's insurance will cover. The patient may be discharged home with a visit from a visiting nurse later the same day to evaluate the patient's need for these services and to make arrangements for him or her in the home. An individual may be discharged home only when certain equipment such as a hospital-style bed and oxygen has been delivered to the home. If a patient feels he or she is being discharged before he or she is ready, the patient can file a complaint with the hospital.

A follow-up from the hospital staff, either physician, nurse, or case manager, should take place within two weeks of discharge to review the results of any tests that were done in the hospital that came in after the patient was discharged, to remind the patient of the follow-up appointment with the physician, to see if the patient has any questions about any new medications that were added in the hospital, and to be sure that no problems arose after discharge that have not been addressed. Such follow-up calls help to ensure a successful recovery.

DISCHARGE PLANNING AND PROCEDURE

There are intended to be fundamental principles applying to discharge from hospital. Unfortunately they are frequently disregarded. Discharge is only meant to happen when:

i. Key decisions have been made about the provision of any care required and the source of that care agreed.

ii. Funding of all needed resources or accommodation after discharge has been established.

Discharge from hospital should be planned and arranged by a team which will include, or have links with, Social Services and Health (the PCT). There may be a specific member of Hospital staff acting as a Discharge Facilitator (or co-ordinator).

The Patients Charter provides for you and your carer(s) to be consulted at all stages regarding any arrangements made for you. However, there is intense pressure on hospital beds and hospital discharge may not always be correctly organised. If you are funding and arranging your own post-hospital care, the pressure may be particularly acute.

DISCHARGE PROCEDURE

Intermediate care may be available to bridge possible gaps between the services provided by health and social Services. It is designed to help those people leaving hospital, but not able to manage independently in their own homes. It would include physiotherapy and/or occupational therapy, where required. This type of care may be provided in a nursing home, or in a person's own home. It would typically last for six weeks, but local variations will apply.

There are rules and check lists for all aspects of discharge procedure. Here is an outline of what you might expect:

Date of discharge: Patients and carers should be given adequate warning of the precise date and time of leaving hospital. There should be contingency planning for Friday afternoon or weekend discharges.

Identifying Requirements: Appropriate transport should be organised, including an escort if necessary.

Home arrival: The home of a patient living alone should be correctly prepared for their return. Unfortunately, this is often neglected.

Emergencies: The patient should be provided with a hospital contact telephone number in case of medical difficulties following discharge.

Special Needs: The patient and/or carer should be provided with precise information concerning rest, diet, medications and follow-up appointments. This information should be provided in a form appropriate for people from ethnic communities, those with learning disabilities, or those with sensory impairment.

After Care: Support services such as domiciliary care, district nurse or meals on wheels should be initiated or re-established, to start on the needed date. Any necessary home aids and adaptations should be supplied with full use instructions for you and your carer(s).

GP: Written discharge information should be sent to your GP within 24 hours of your leaving hospital. Advice of all follow-up hospital appointments will also be forwarded.

Home Transfer: On-going Care Plans should be provided for all patients transferring to care homes.

Intensive Support/Palliative Care: When necessary, this might entail further inpatient care, placement in a care home, or an intensive support package at home. Palliative care, where people with a life threatening condition no longer respond to medical treatment, also comes into this category.

The diagnosis of life-threatening illness brings with it a transformation of life - where emotional, physical and specific medical needs will need to be met. For those suffering such conditions and their families, it is comforting to know that a wide range of specialist support is available to accommodate changing circumstances and preferences.

From first diagnosis of conditions such as cancer your specialist hospital team, in conjunction with your GP, will be the fulcrum which activates all available aspects and sources of hospital and home care. The objective will be that all your wishes as regards treatment options will be taken into full account at all times - within an appropriate programme for every stage of your condition.

There comes a time, nevertheless, when you may be told that further treatment or surgery will not help. It does not mean that nothing else can, or will be done for you. There will certainly be treatment available that will be able to control the symptoms caused by your deteriorating condition. This type of treatment is termed Palliative Care. It focuses on controlling pain and symptoms - and meeting the social, emotional and spiritual needs of you and your family.

CARE OF THE UNIT AFTER DISCHARGE

Palliative care may be provided by home care nurses, doctors or other health professionals from voluntary or hospices or specialist Palliative Care Units and a wide range of other voluntary and statutory services.

These professionals are highly skilled, widely experienced and sympathetic in managing patients' needs and changing circumstances. Palliative care can be provided in your own home, a care home, in a hospital or, indeed, in a hospice.

Eventually, someone whose illness is becoming progressively worse may need 24 hour attention and care, may be offered a place in a Hospice - where the objective will be to provide the most appropriate care, all necessary medications and, with that, the very best quality of life. Hospice staff are specially trained to advise on pain and symptom control and to give emotional support to patients, their families and loved ones - during illness and after bereavement.

Intermediate Care: Intermediate care is targeted at people who would otherwise face unnecessarily long hospitals stays, or inappropriate admission to acute hospital care or long term residential care.

Intermediate Care is varied to suit your needs and could involve active therapy, medical treatment or the support of your recovery time. Many of us might understand the whole notion better by thinking of a traditional 'convalescence' provision.

Intermediate Care will be provided with an objective in mind - such as enabling you to resume living independently at home. The plan will be reviewed within a six week period and then decisions made concerning possible longer term rehabilitation needs, or specific home care.

REFERENCES

Aiken, L. H., & Gwyther, M. (1995). Medicare funding of nursing education: The case for policy change. Journal of the American Medical Association, 273, 19

Buerhaus, P. I., Staiger, D. O., & Auerbach, D. I. (2000). Implication of an aging registered nurse workforce. Journal of the American Medical Association, 283(22), 2948–2954.

Burns, N., & Grove, S. (2000). The practice of nursing research (4th ed.). Philadelphia: Saunders. Canadian Association of University Schools of Nursing. (1998).

Carper, B. A. (1978). Fundamental patterns of knowing in nursing. Advances in Nursing Science, 1, 13–23.

Carper, B. A. (1992). Philosophical inquiry in nursing: An application. In J. F. Kikuchi & H. Simmons (Eds.), Philosophic inquiry in nursing. Newbury Park, CA: Sage.

Daley, B. J. (1996). Concept maps: Linking nursing theory to clinical nursing practice. Journal of Continuing Education in Nursing, 27(1), 17–27.

Frik, S. M., Speed, D. J., & Pollock, S. E. (1996). A special pathway for registered nurses with baccalaureate degrees in fields other than nursing. Journal of Nursing Education, 35(4), 152–156.

Hinshaw, A. S., Feetham, S. L., Shaver, J. L. (1999). Handbook of clinical nursing research. Thousand Oaks, CA: Sage.

Lindeman, C. A. (2000). The future of nursing education. Journal of Nursing Education, 39(1), 5–12.

4

Nurse Patient Relationship

The meaning of the word "communication" is at once both clear and obscure. It is clear enough in conventional usage, but obscure when we seek to determine the limits of its application. To illustrate, if someone talks to another and common understanding results (indicated by mutually satisfactory action), we have no qualms about saying that communication has occurred. If, nevertheless, misunderstanding results (indicated by mutually unsatisfactory action), we are uncertain whether we should say that there has been poor, or no, communication. Further, if someone does not talk to another and the latter as a result gains certain impressions of the former, has communication occurred?

The problem is familiar. It seems impossible to draw a line between those situations that we conventionally term "communication" and those we do not, short of a purely arbitrary distinction. And the many and varied definitions of "communication" appearing in the literature of various fields of study often appear, at first glance at least, to compound the difficulty.

MEANING OF COMMUNICATION

We must be concerned about defining communication. Certainly our notion of this process determines to no small degree our approach to speech training, how broadly or narrowly we view our subject, how we relate it to other areas of study. To accomplish our intention, we shall present a number of definitions of "communication" in a two-fold classification and examine the application of these definitions to a series of situations in which human responses and interactions occur. Such classification and application should give us some insights into the problem of definition, into the relationship among existing definitions, and provide us with the perspective necessary to select the most fundamental, consistent, and useful definition of "communication," and to see its relationship to the process of speech.

LEVELS

Phatic Communication: Using conventional messages to establish rapport, to break the ice, and/or to end a conversation. We expect phatic communication at the beginning and end of every conversation, regardless of our feelings about an individual.

Factual communication: Using events, making observations, offering knowledge to others in a manner which can be called chit chat or small talk. Factual communication is relatively safe and most do this well.

Evaluative communication: Offering opinions, ideas and judgments to others. It's significant to consider the value of critical and creative thinking, as well as the relational meanings of messages that are exchanged. When using evaluative communication, consider carefully the significance of descriptive, provisional, and accountable expressions. Strive to avoid cautionary language, sarcasm, and nonverbal put-downs (e.g., rolling your eyes in response to another's comments).

Gut-level communication involves sharing our emotions and feelings with another. We are sharing our very essence when we allow others to know our heart. This is risky business! Societies place constraints upon the specific emotions which can be conveyed (e.g., It's good to express love; it's bad to express hatred). We also have rules about when and how feelings can be expressed ("That was the wrong time and place for arguing with your spouse.")

Peak communication: Coming together with another in an extraordinary way. Two persons who are gut levelling experience a transformation when they are sharing the exact same emotion with the same level of intensity. This is also called, "communal-level communication."

ELEMENTS

Approach: Timing of communication; choice of medium; tone and point of view (perspective, attitude, and relationship regarding audience, intention, and material); recognition of audience (reader vs. writer orientation); direct vs. indirect presentation (ordering of evidence and conclusions); persuasive strategies and rhetorical appeals (logos, pathos, ethos)

Checkpoints:

- Timing and choice of medium are appropriate to the intention, audience, and material.
- Tone is appropriate to the intention, audience, and material.
- Material is made relevant to the reader (reader's interests and concerns are recognized).
- Conclusions are presented directly (conclusion first, evidence last) to a sympathetic audience, indirectly (evidence first, conclusion last) to a unsympathetic or hostile audience.
- Persuasive strategy incorporates a mixture of rhetorical approaches (appeals to logic, feelings, and ethics or credibility).

Development: Organization (logical arrangement and sequence); evidence and support (relevance, specificity, accuracy and sufficiency of detail); knowledge of subject and material; quality of perception, analysis, and insight

Main points:

- Material is arranged in a logical and coherent sequence.
- Conclusion or closing restates the argument and identifies the action to be taken.
- Examples are relevant, specific, detailed, sufficient, and persuasive.
- Quotations support the argument.
- Handling of material demonstrates knowledge and insight.

Clarity: Presentation of thesis or central argument (statement of intention, delineation or narrowing of topic, relevance of subordinate or secondary arguments); word choice; technical language and jargon; structure (sentence, paragraph, document); coherence devices (organizational statement, repetition of words and phrases, progression from familiar to unfamiliar, topic and transitional sentences); textual markers (headings, highlighting, formatting features)

Main points:

- Purpose or central idea is sufficiently limited for meaningful discussion.
- Purpose or central idea is stated clearly, commonly in the opening.

- Organizational statement is offered, commonly at the end of the opening.
- Subordinate ideas are effectively identified and related clearly to the main intention or central idea.
- Language is clear, specific, accurate, and appropriate to the audience, intention, and material.
- Word choice is clear, specific, accurate, unassuming, and free of clichés and misused jargon.
- Technical language and terms are defined and explained as required (depending on knowledge of the audience).
- Sentences are free of ambiguity.
- Text is coherent, with new information linked to previously discussed information (ordered within sentences as "something old/something new").
- Transitions between paragraphs are clear and helpful.
- Text is appropriately highlighted (bullets, paragraphing, boldface, italics, underlining, etc.) to engage the reader and reinforce the main points.

Style: Word choice (economy, precision, and specificity of language and detail; abstract vs. concrete language; action verbs vs. linking or weak verbs with nominalizations; figures of speech: schemes and tropes); tone (personality and humor); active vs. passive voice; sentence variety

Main points:

- Word choice is economical, clear, specific, accurate, unassuming, and free of clichés and misused jargon.
- Action verbs are preferred over weak verbs with nominalizations (as in recommend over make a recommendation).
- Language is appropriately concrete or abstract (signifying or not signifying things that can be perceived by the senses).
- Figurative language (metaphors and similes, as well as other tropes and schemes) enrich and deepen the argument.
- Active voice is preferred over passive voice (active voice is used to emphasize the performer of the action; passive voice is used to emphasize the receiver of the action).
- Sentences are free of wordiness and unnecessarily complex constructions.

- Variety in sentence structure and sentence length creates emphasis.

Correctness: Rules and conventions of spelling, grammar, punctuation, usage, and idiom; style (appropriateness of word choice and level of formality to audience, intention, and material); social and cultural appropriateness; accuracy in proofreading

Main points:

- Spelling (including technical terms and proper names) is correct.
- Correct words are used to convey the intended meaning.
- Rules of grammar and syntax are followed, including pronoun-noun agreement, subject-verb agreement, appropriate verb tense, pronoun case, possessive forms, parallel construction, etc.

TYPES OF COMMUNICATION

Communication can occur via various processes and methods and depending on the channel used and the style of communication there can be various types of communication.

Types of Communication Based on Communication Channels

Based on the channels used for communicating, the process of communication can be broadly classified as verbal communication and non-verbal communication. Verbal communication includes written and oral communication whereas the non-verbal communication includes body language, facial expressions and visuals diagrams or pictures used for communication.

- Verbal Communication: Verbal communication is further divided into written and oral communication. The oral communication refers to the spoken words in the communication process. Oral communication can either be face-to-face communication or a conversation over the phone or on the voice chat over the Internet. Spoken conversations or dialogs are influenced by voice modulation, pitch, volume and even the speed and clarity of speaking. The other type of verbal communication is written communication. Written communication can be either via snail mail, or email. The effectiveness of written communication depends on the style of writing, vocabulary used, grammar, clarity and precision of language.

- Nonverbal Communication: Non-verbal communication includes the overall body language of the person who is speaking, which will include the body posture, the hand gestures, and overall body movements. The facial expressions also play a major role while communication since the expressions on a person's face say a lot about his/her mood. On the other hand gestures like a handshake, a smile or a hug can independently convey emotions. Non verbal communication can also be in the form of pictorial representations, signboards, or even photographs, sketches and paintings.

Types of Communication Based on Style and Purpose

Based on the style of communication, there can be two broad categories of communication, which are formal and informal communication that have their own set of characteristic features.

- Formal Communication: Formal communication includes all the instances where communication has to occur in a set formal format. Typically this can include all sorts of business communication or corporate communication. The style of communication in this form is very formal and official. Official conferences, meetings and written memos and corporate letters are used for communication. Formal communication can also occur between two strangers when they meet for the first time. Hence formal communication is straightforward, official and always precise and has a stringent and rigid tone to it.
- Informal Communication: Informal communication includes instances of free unrestrained communication between people who share a casual rapport with each other. Informal communication requires two people to have a similar wavelength and hence occurs between friends and family. Informal communication does not have any rigid rules and guidelines. Informal conversations need not necessarily have boundaries of time, place or even subjects for that matter since we all know that friendly chats with our loved ones can simply go on and on.

PROCESS OF COMMUNICATION

Communication can best be summarized as the transmission of a message from a sender to a receiver in an understandable manner. The significance of effective communication is immeasurable in the world of business and in personal life. From a business perspective, effective communication is an absolute must, because it usually accounts for the difference between success and failure or profit and loss. It has become clear that effective business communication is critical to the successful operation of modern enterprise. Every business individual needs to understand the fundamentals of effective communication.

Effective communication is the most critical component of total quality management. The manner in which persons perceive and talk to each other at work about different issues is a major determinant of the business success. It has proven been proven that poor communication reduces quality, weakens productivity, and eventually leads to anger and a lack of trust among persons within the organization.

Feedback is the final link in the chain of the communication process. After receiving a message, the receiver responds in some way and signals that response to the sender. The signal may take the form of a spoken comment, a long sigh, a written message, a smile, or some other action. Without feedback, the sender cannot confirm that the receiver has interpreted the message properly.

Successful and effective communication within an organization stems from the implementation of the communication process. All members within an organization will improve their communication skills if they follow the communication process, and stay away from the different barriers. It has been proven that persons that understand the communication process will blossom into more effective communicators, and effective communicators have a greater opportunity for becoming a success.

METHODS OF EFFECTIVE COMMUNICATION

Effective communication is not just a business skill - it is a life skill & the most significant source of personal power at work, family & social situations. Communication is the process of understanding and being understood through ideas, facts, thoughts and emotions. Good communication is determined not by how well we say things but by how well we have been understood.

Listening skill is as significant to effective communication as is speaking skill. Though some people are very good listeners, many unfortunately, are poor listeners. Listening skill is concerned with concentration and the ability to perceive the proper significance and relationship among the speaker's ideas. Real or genuine listening cannot be faked. To do it one must be what is called fully present by participating physically, mentally and emotionally.

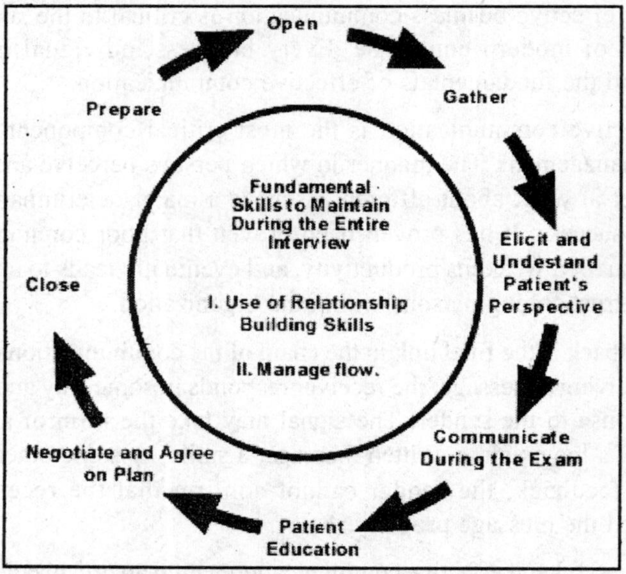

Fig. Effective Communication

ATTENDING SKILLS

- Attending Skills: Listening actively by maintaining eye contact, clarifying understanding, exploring in an open-ended manner, addressing feelings.
- Responding: Conveying genuine interest, expressing open acceptance in a non-judgmental manner
- Facilitating: Expressing honest feedback and offering encouragement.
- Clarification: Statements or questions used to gain further information about how the developing teacher is thinking.
- Perception Checking: Statement or questions used to gain further information about the developing teacher is responding emotionally.
- Empathy: Statements that identify with and express understanding of the feelings, situation or motives of the developing teacher.
- Concrete Examples: Statements that refer to specific events, behaviours or provide specific instances of observed behaviours.

RAPPORT BUILDING SKILLS

In rapport building following points should be considered:

- Conversations should be a balanced two-way flow of dialogue.
- It's good to initiate conversations with small talk.
- It's good to call people by name whenever possible. It makes a good, lasting impression, and it makes the other individual feel significant and special.
- Regular use of these courtesy words and phrases is significant to show politeness and build rapport.
- Smiling when greeting people and at appropriate times greatly helps build rapport.
- Making eye contact is significant for building rapport. It gives the impression you're interested and engaged in the conversation, and you have good self-confidence.
- Communicating at eye level helps build rapport.
- It's best to bring the conversation to an end by making a polite closing comment or gesture.
- Never say anything that might hurt or offend the individual.
- Showing empathy (sensitivity) to another person's feelings helps build rapport.

EMPATHY

Empathetic listening involves more than understanding the words that are said. You listen with your ears but also, more significantly listen with your eyes and with your heart. You listen for feeling, you listen for meaning, and you listen for behaviour.

HELPING RELATIONSHIPS (NPR)

Nurses are accountable for evaluating, planning, implementing, and assessing nursing care for an identified group of patients. Nurses collaborate with all members of the interdisciplinary team. Nurses have the authority to make decisions within the scope of their practice and to advocate on behalf of their patients. They prioritize patient care needs and are responsible for nursing care outcomes. The nurse develops therapeutic relationships with patients and families. This professional nurse-patient relationship exists whether it's through a single interaction, a shift, or an entire length of stay on a unit, or throughout the Health System. Scheduling of personnel and time develops the nurse-patient relationship.

Patient assignments are determined collaboratively on each shift, and decisions are made based on patient needs, patient acuity, and Resident Nurse level of competency and experience. Every effort is made to maximize continuity of care and caregiver in order to achieve an optimal therapeutic relationship. Nurse Managers assure adequate resources to meet patient needs based on unit census, patient acuity, and overall activity within the respective units. The nurse retains ultimate accountability for the process and outcomes of care. Delegation by nurses is based on patient needs, complexity of care, competency of the individual accepting the delegation, and the timing of the care to be given. The care provider receiving a delegated assignment from a nurse accepts duty, authority and accountability of the work assigned.

Communication between all members of the health care team is essential to the achievement of optimal patient outcomes. Nurses collaborate with the patient and important others as well as other members of the healthcare team to identify specific patient needs. Acting as a patient advocate, the nurse communicates these needs directly and proactively to the interdisciplinary team. Integrating information and coordinating all aspects of patient care are the roles and duties of the professional nurse.

DIMENSIONS OF HELPING RELATIONSHIP

Nurses should be able to answer the questions of the patients. Awareness helps the nurse to be honest and avoid the unethical use of patients to meet the personal needs.

- Value systems: Values are notions that are formed as result of life experience with family, friends, culture, education, work and relaxation. Value systems provide the framework for many daily decisions and actions. By being aware of value systems, nurses can identify situations in which value systems are in conflict. Many therapeutic relationships test the nurse's values. E.g. A patient may describe a sexual behaviour that the nurse finds unacceptable; a patient may talk about the divorce where as the nurse may strongly believe that marriage contracts should not be broken; or a patient may be religious but the nurse may not believe in God or religion.
- Value clarification Process: It allows the individual to discover their values by evaluating, exploring and determining what those values are and what priority they hold in decision making process. Seven criteria are used to determine the value. These

criteria should be considered in relation to a person's strongest value and tested against the persons own definition of a value.

The three criteria of choosing relay on the persons cognitive abilities, the two criteria of prizing emphasize the emotional or affective level, and the two criteria of acting have a behavioural focus.

- The mature valuing process: It is complex. There is no guarantee that the choice made will prove to be self -actualizing. The valuing process in the mature individual has the following characteristics:
- It is fluid and flexible
- The valuing experience is tied to a particular time and experience
- Personal experience provides the value information
- Exploration of feelings: The nurses should be open to, aware of and in control of their feelings so that they can be used to help the patient. The feelings that the nurse have serve a significant intention. In helping others, nurses have many feelings; elation at seeing a patient improves., disappointment when a patient regresses, distress when a patient refuses the help, anger when a patient is demanding or manipulative and power when a patient express strong dependence on the nurse
- Serving as a role model: A nurse has an obligation to model maladaptive and growth producing behaviour. If a nurse has a chaotic personal life, it will show in the nurse's work with patients, decreasing the effectiveness of care. The effective nurse has a fulfilling and satisfying personal life that is not dominated by conflict, distress, or denial and that the nurses approach to life conveys a sense of growing, hopefulness, and adapting.
- Altruism: Altruism is concern for the welfare of others. It does not mean that an altruistic individual should not expect adequate compensation and recognition or must practice denial or self sacrifice. A sense of altruism also can apply to changing social conditions to meet human welfare needs. One goal of all helping professional should be to create a people -serving and growth facilitating society. So the necessary goal of nurse is to work to change the larger structure and process of society in ways that will promote the persons health and well-being.
- Ethics and duty: Nurse's sense of ethics is the need to assume duty for behaviour. This involves knowing limitations and

strengths and being responsible for them. As a member of health team nurse has ready access to the knowledge and expertise of other people; these resources should be used appropriately.

ACTION DIMENSIONS

The action oriented conditions for facilitative interpersonal relationship are confrontation, immediacy, therapist self disclosure.catharsis and role play.

Confrontation: It is an expression by the nurse of perceived discrepancies in the patient's behaviour. The three categories of confrontation are listed in the following:

- Discrepancies between the patient's expressions of what she or he is and what he or she wants to be.
- Discrepancies' between the patient's verbal self expression and nonverbal behaviour.
- Discrepancies between the patient's verbal expressed experience of himself or herself and the nurses experience of him or her.

Confrontation is an attempt to by the nurse to make the patient aware of incongruence in his or her feelings, attitudes, beliefs and behaviours. It also may lead to the discovery of ambivalent feelings in the patient. It is not limited to negative aspects of the patient. It includes pointing out discrepancies involving resources and strengths that are unrecognized and unused. It requires that the nurse collect sufficient data about the patient's history and accumulate sufficient perception and observations of verbal and nonverbal communication so that validation of reality is possible. The nurse must have developed an understanding of the patient to perceive discrepancies, inconsistencies in the word and deed, distortions and defences. The nurse must be willing and able to work through the crisis after confronting the patient. Without this commitment confrontation lacks therapeutic potential and can be damaging to both patient and nurse.

Timing in relationship: Before confrontation nurse should evaluate the following components:

- The trust level in the relationship
- The timing
- The patients stress level
- The strength of the patient's defence mechanisms.
- The patients perceived need for personal space or closeness

- The patients level of rage and tolerance for hearing another perception

PATIENT TEACHING

A newly admitted patient is surrounded by shocked and confused family members, all of them attempting to cope with the impact of his new diagnosis. It could be diabetes mellitus, stroke, or TB infection. He may have fallen, and family members question his ability to recover from a hip fracture. Or it may be surgery for colon cancer that triggers the feelings of fear and uncertainty. Whatever the circumstances, the chances of his return to a quality life rest to a great extent on the teaching skills of his nurses. In fact, patient education is now considered central to achieving effective outcomes for patients and is often recognized in state practice acts as a legal duty of nurses.

One of the most significant roles of nurses is that of patient advocate, reflecting their ability to protect the interests of patients who cannot represent themselves because of illness or inadequate health knowledge. Inherent in the role of advocate, then, is the role of teacher, and there's a place for patient education in virtually every aspect of nursing care. Some nurses serve exclusively as educators for special groups such as patients with diabetes or breast cancer. However, the nurse at the bedside in the medical-surgical setting is often the one whose bond with the patient leads him to feel comfortable in asking about his health experience.

Fast discharges and the use of sophisticated medical devices at home can be a dangerous combination for your patient. To keep him safe and his recovery on track, use these suggestions.

GENERAL GUIDELINES

Adults learn on a need to know basis-for instance, they need to know how to solve a problem, acquire a new skill, or meet a personal goal. In the hospital, they're commonly motivated to learn what they need to know so they can take care of themselves. So when the Nurse teaches the patient, she should emphasize why this information will be useful to him.

The Nurse should keep in mind that a patient may need time to cope with a new diagnosis. He may be experiencing overwhelming feelings of grief, powerlessness, fear, and vulnerability. So you may need to talk about his feelings before you start teaching and follow up with him afterward to make sure his emotions didn't interfere with learning.

Use fundamental learning principles: Involve the patient in learning, base new knowledge on previous knowledge and experience, and give him the opportunity to repeat skills.

Plan an uninterrupted time for teaching. Post a sign on the patient's door or take him to a conference room. Make sure the environment is comfortable.

PROCESS

The Teaching-Learning Process includes: the teaching process, patient evaluation, identifying the learning need, setting learning objectives, defining teaching methods and assessing the teaching outcome. Learning is a change in behaviours such as knowledge, skills, beliefs and attitudes. Learning is an ongoing, life-long process and not a one-time encounter. For learning to be sustained, it takes continuous reinforcement. Individuals must be ready, willing and able to learn.

The individual patient's learning need determines the teaching process. The family or important others should be included in the plan. This process should be documented in a written teaching plan.

- The content - What is to be taught
- The method - How it is taught
- Learning - The teaching/learning objective
- Testing - How learning is evaluated

Patient Assessment

Learning occurs in three, interrelated areas: cognitive, psychomotor and affective. It's significant to evaluate the patient's readiness to learn in these three areas before creating a teaching plan.

Cognitive or intellectual skills require knowing, thinking and remembering. It's helpful for the nurse to ask: What is the patient's reading level? What is the patient's highest level of schooling completed? Can he understand language? If not, what languages, does he speak? Is he oriented to time, place and person? How is the patient's memory? How will the patient's intellectual abilities affect his ability to learn, understand, apply new information and recall it later? Is he too sick or distressed to learn at this time?

Psychomotor skills are physical skills, which require integrating both mental and muscular activity. It's helpful for the nurse to ask: How is the patient's hearing and sight? Is the patient able to write? Is his mobility impaired by an amputation, stroke or other disability? Is he able to perform fine motor tasks with his hands?

Affective involves beliefs, values and attitudes. It's helpful for the nurse to ask: Is the patient motivated to learn and change his behaviour? Can the team identify the barriers to learning and address them so successful learning can take place? Does the patient recognize the need to learn? How do the patient's values from his social and cultural background influence his motivation to learn? Can he be an active participant in learning through listening, learning and non-verbal communication? Is he anxious? Is the patient distracted by his environment?

ROLE OF NURSE AND INTEGRATING TEACHING IN NURSING PROCESS

The significance of education and teaching as vital components of the nursing process has been recognized since the early days of the profession. However, the central role of nurses in providing patient education is especially accentuated in the dialysis setting where the patients spend large amounts of time getting treatments, with many opportunities for planned as well as spontaneous teaching.

The nursing process provides a method for individualizing patient care and education for each patient and event. The first step in this process is a nursing evaluation: the process of collecting data to identify the needs and problems of an individual patient and family. In the evaluation process, the nurse collects information from various sources, validates this information, sorts and categorizes data, and summarizes or interprets it. The end product: a nursing diagnosis of educational need: is a judgment based on sound data and information.

Many healthcare professionals have the misconception that evaluation is a prolonged, time intensive process. However, in many cases nurses perform evaluations instinctively on a day to-day basis. In this brief scenario, the nurse has applied the principles of evaluation by integrating physical symptoms, a brief interview with the patient, and knowledge of the patient's history and laboratory data to detect a clinical challenge.

REFERENCES

Aiken, L. H. (1995). Transformation of the nursing workforce. Nursing Outlook, 43(5), 201–209.

Baker, C. M. (1994). School health: Policy issues. Nursing and Health Care, 15(4), 178–184.

Boccuzzi, N. K. (1998). CAPNA: Columbia Advanced Practice Nurse Associates: Advanced practice nurses found a landmark practice. American Journal of Nursing, 98(11), 34–35.

Chamberlain, P., Chen, Y., Osuna, E., & Yamamoto, C. (1995). Innovative culture shock prescribed for health care. Nursing Outlook, 43(5), 232–234.

Economic Policy Institute. (1999). Sharing care: The changing nature of nursing. Washington, DC: Author.

Falter, E. J. (1999). The health care continuum. American Journal of Nursing, 99(1), 63–64.

Feldstein, P. J. (1993). Health care economics (4th ed.). Albany, NY: Delmar Publishers.

Friedman, E. (1994). The uninsured: From dilemma to crisis. In P. Lee & C. Estes (Eds.), The nation's health (4th ed.). Boston: Jones & Bartlett.

Grace, H. K. (1994). Can medical costs be contained? In J. C. McCloskey, & H. K. Grace (Eds.), Current issues in nursing (4th ed.). St. Louis: Mosby-Yearbook.

Harrison, B. S., Faircloth, J. W., & Yaryan, L. (1995). The impact of legislation on the role of the school nurse. Nursing Outlook, 43(2), 57–61.

5

Process of Nursing

The nursing process is a process by which nurses deliver care to patients, supported by nursing models or philosophies. The nursing process was originally an adapted form of problem-solving and is classified as a deductive theory.

The nursing process is a cyclical and ongoing process that can end at any stage if the problem is solved. The nursing process exists for every problem that the patient has, and for every element of patient care, rather than once for each patient. The nurse's assessment of care will lead to changes in the implementation of the care and the patient's needs are likely to change during their stay in hospital as their health either improves or deteriorates. The nursing process not only focuses on ways to improve the patient's physical needs, but also on social and emotional needs as well.

- Cyclic and dynamic
- Goal directed and client centred
- Interpersonal and collaborative
- Universally applicable
- Systematic

The nursing process is not something foreign or unusually complex. On the contrary, we use the nursing process method on a daily basis without even realizing it. For instance, a trip to the gas station to get fuel requires evaluating the various prices and the number of people waiting to get gas among other things. A subsequent decision, or diagnosis, is made based on the former criteria. This may include pulling into the gas station to fuel up or going down the road for better prices and/or less of a crowd. The price is right and there's not much of a crowd, we're pulling in. Now the Planning can take place. This may include which pump to use, how much gas to put in the tank, whether or not to clean the windows along with other things. We're at the pump and ready to fuel up. We must now implement what we planned prior to pulling up to the pump. We've pulled up on the passenger side because the gas tank resides on this side, part of our plan. We've also given ourselves enough room to exit without getting blocked in by another vehicle, part of our plan also. We now unscrew the gas cap and begin fuelling or Implementing what we planned. Things went well. We are fuelled up and have exited the gas station without complication. Our Assessment of the trip to the gas station would be a good one. We may choose to use this method in the future. The Nursing process is that simple in theory. However, as a nurse, the nursing process tool will be used for more complex and difficult situations but is applied the same way as the gas station analogy.

The nursing process involves skills a nurse should possess when he or she has to initiate the initial phase of the process. Having these skills contributes to the greater improvement of the nurse's delivery of health care to the patient, including the patient's level of health, or health status.

- Cognitive or Intellectual skills, such as analyzing the problem, problem solving, critical thinking and making judgements regarding the patient's needs. Included in these skills are the ability to identify, differentiate actual and potential health problems through observation and decision making by synthesizing nursing knowledge previously acquired.
- Interpersonal skills, which includes therapeutic communication, active listening, conveying knowledge and information, developing trust or rapport-building with the patient, and ethically obtaining required and relevant information from the patient which is then to be utilized in health problem formulation and analysis.
- Technical skills, which includes knowledge and skills required to correctly and safely manipulate and handle appropriate equipment required by the patient in performing medical or diagnostic procedures, such as vital signs, and medication administrations.

The following are the steps or phases of the nursing process.

- Assessment (of patient's needs)
- Diagnosis (of human response needs that nurses can deal with)
- Planning (of patient's care)

- Implementation (of care)
- Assessment (of the success of the implemented care)

CRITICAL THINKING AND NURSING JUDGEMENT

The significance of critical thinking in nursing is so evident that educational programs are evaluated according to the development of skills related to this sort of thinking. Numerous authors have underscored the need for nurses to be able to think critically in order to use the appropriate knowledge and skilled judgments in delivering patient care.

In this regard, several definitions have been postulated to describe various and profound aspects of critical thinking in general and within the profession of nursing in particular. Critical thinking is a composite of attitudes, knowledge, and skills which includes:

- Attitudes of inquiry that involve an ability to recognize the existence of problems and an acceptance of the general need for evidence in support of what is asserted to be true;
- Knowledge of the nature of valid inferences, abstractions, and generalizations in which the weight or accuracy of different kinds of evidence are logically determined; and
- Skills in applying and applying the above attitudes and knowledge.

Habits of the mind of critical thinking in nursing include confidence, contextual perspective, creativity, flexibility, inquisitiveness, intellectual integrity, intuition, open-mindedness, perseverance, and reflection. Skills of critical thinking in nursing consist of analyzing, applying standards, discriminating, information seeking, and logical reasoning, predicting and transforming knowledge. Varied perspectives of critical thinking exist in nursing.

CRITICAL THINKING: THINKING AND LEARNING

Critical thinking is the disciplined, intellectual process of employing adept reasoning as a guide to belief or action. In nursing, critical thinking for clinical decision-making is the ability to think in a systematic and logical manner with openness to question and reflect on the reasoning process used to ensure safe nursing practice and quality care. Critical thinking when developed in the practitioner includes adherence to intellectual standards, proficiency in using reasoning, a obligation to develop and maintain intellectual traits of the mind and habits of thought and the competent use of thinking skills and abilities for sound clinical judgements and safe decision-making.

Practitioners in nursing who are critical thinkers value and adhere to intellectual standards. Critical thinkers strive to be clear, accurate, precise, logical complete, significant and fair when they listen, speak, read and write. Critical thinkers think deeply and broadly. Their thinking is adequate for their intended intention. All thinking can be examined in light of these standards and as we reflect on the quality of our thinking we begin to recognize when we are being unclear, imprecise, vague or inaccurate. As nurses, we want to eradicate irrelevant, inconsistent and illogical thoughts as we reason about client care. Nurses use language to clearly communicate in-depth information that is significant to nursing care. Nurses are not focused on the trivial or irrelevant. Nurses who are critical thinkers hold all their views and reasoning to these standards as well as, the claims of others such that the quality of nurse's thinking improves over time thus eliminating confusion and ambiguity in the presentation and understanding of thoughts and ideas.

Reasoning in nursing involves eight elements of thought. Critical thinking involves trying to figure out something; a problem, an issue, the views of another person, a theory or an idea. To figure things out we need to enter into the thinking of the other individual and then to comprehend as best we can the structure of their thinking. This also applies to our own thinking as well.

Critical inquiry is a significant quality for safe practice. Nurses must pose questions about practice and be willing to attempt to seek answers about practice. Nurses must be willing to attempt to seek answers to the difficult questions inherent in practice, as well as the obvious. Question posing presupposes intellectual humility and a disposition to admit to one's areas of ignorance as well as, intellectual curiosity and perseverance and willingness to seek answers. Critical thinkers in nursing are truth seekers and demonstrate open-mindedness and tolerance for others' views with constant sensitivity to the possibility of their own bias.

Nurse's who are critical thinkers value intellectually challenging situations and are self-confident in their well reasoned thoughts. To reason effectively, nurses have developed skills and abilities essential for sound reasoning.

NURSING PROCESS OVERVIEW

The nursing process is a problem-solving approach that enables the nurse to provide care in an organized scientific manner. The goal of the nursing process is to alleviate, minimize, or prevent actual or potential health problems. The nursing process can be applied in any interaction that involves a nurse and a client. The process can take place in a variety of settings, including a hospital, community setting, private home, or long term care facility. The following are the steps or phases of the nursing process.

- Assessment (of patient's needs)
- Diagnosis (of human response needs that nurses can deal with)
- Planning (of patient's care)
- Implementation (of care)
- Evaluation (of the success of the implemented care)

ASSESSMENT

The nurse collects data about the health status of the client. The data is subjective and objective. Subjective data is commonly documented in the clients own words. This data includes such things as previous experiences, and sensations or emotions that only the client can describe. The Objective data is obtained by the health team, through observation, physical examination, or/and diagnostic testing. Objective data can be seen or measured. Sources of subjective data and objective data are the client, the family and significant others, medical records, and other health care team members.

Assessment includes, the Health History and Physical Evaluation. The health history is a collection of subjective data that includes information on both the client's past and present health status. It is used in conjunction with the physical examination and laboratory findings as a basis for drawing conclusions about an individual's state of health. It allows positive aspects, health problems, health habits as well as abnormal symptoms, health problems, health teaching needs, and health concerns to be identified.

The following nursing models are used to gather the necessary and relevant information from the patient in order to effectively deliver quality nursing care. This will help the nurse determine the ranking of the problems encountered.

- Gordon's functional health patterns
- Roy's adaptation model
- Body systems model
- Maslow's hierarchy of needs

Components of a Comprehensive Health History

- Date history obtained.
- Source of history.
- Interpreter if used.
- Reason for seeking health care.
- Client Profile Data.
- Present Illness Data.
- Present Health Status.
- Past Personal data.
- Family Medical data.
- Life-style data.
- Health Management data.
- Psychological data.
- Review of Systems.

Physical Assessment

Physical evaluation can be broken down into four components;

Inspection

Inspection is the visual examination of the client.

Palpation

Palpation uses the sense of touch to evaluate various parts of the body and helps to confirm findings that are noted on inspection. The hands, especially the finger tips are used to evaluate skin temperature, check pulses, texture, moisture, masses, tenderness, or pain. Ask the Client for permission first and explain to your client what you intend to examine. Establish client trust with being professional. Please remember to use warm hands. Any tender areas should be palpated last.

Percussion

Percussion is the striking of the body surface with short, sharp strokes in order to produce palpable vibrations and characteristic sounds. It is used to determine the location, size, shape, and density of underlying structures; to detect the presences of air or fluid in a body space; and to elicit tenderness.

Auscultation

Auscultation is listening to sounds developed inside the body. These include breath sounds, heart sounds, vascular sounds, and bowel sounds. It is used to detect the presence of normal and abnormal sounds and to evaluate them in terms of loudness, pitch, quality, frequency and duration.

NURSING DIAGNOSIS

The nursing diagnosis is derived from data gathered during the evaluation. Health problems or potential health problems are identified and formulated into nursing diagnosis. Nursing Diagnosis is the basis for planning nursing interventions that help prevent, minimize or alleviate specific health issues.

A Medical Diagnosis is much different than nursing diagnosis, it is used to define etiology of the disease. It only focuses is on the function and malfunction of a specific organ system. The two are very different.

A Nursing Diagnosis is written in a format called "PES".

- P stands for Problem
- E stands for Etiology or cause of problem
- S stands Signs and Symptoms of problem

By using all of the components of the nursing diagnosis, the problem is clearly communicated to everyone involved in the clients care.

Types of Diagnosis

- Actual diagnosis: A statement about a health problem that the client has and the benefit from nursing care. An example of an actual nursing diagnosis is: Ineffective airway clearance related to decreased energy as manifested by an ineffective cough.
- Risk diagnosis: A statement about health problems that a client doesn't have yet, but is at a higher than normal risk of developing in the near future. An example of a risk diagnosis is: Risk for injury related to altered mobility and disorientation.
- Possible diagnosis: A statement about a health problem that the client might have now, but the nurse doesn't yet have enough information to make an actual diagnosis. An example of a possible diagnosis is: Possible fluid volume deficit related to frequent vomiting for three days as manifested by increased pulse rate.

- Syndrome diagnosis: Used when a cluster of nursing diagnoses are seen together. An example of a syndrome diagnosis is: Rape-trauma syndrome related to anxiety about potential health problems as manifested by anger, genitourinary discomfort, and sleep pattern disturbance.
- Wellness diagnosis: Describes an aspect of the client that is at a low level of wellness. An example of a wellness diagnosis is: Potential for enhanced organized infant behaviour, related to prematurity and as manifested by response to visual and auditory stimuli.

PLANNING

The planning phase of the Nursing Process involves the development of a nursing care plan for the client based on the nursing diagnosis. The nursing care plan is a communication tool used by Nurses to care for their clients. Care plans that are kept up to date are vital tools to provide continuity of care, prevent complications and provide for health teaching and discharge planning. Goals should be stated in terms of client outcomes. Nursing outcomes examples are: Skin and Mucous Membranes, Wound Healing, Primary Intention, and Urinary Continence. Each of these nursing sensitive outcomes is labelled, defined, and includes criteria for the evaluating the status of the outcome over time.

Nursing orders are the actions for interventions prescribed to help achieve the stated goals and objectives. When writing nursing orders remember to include:

- What
- Where
- When
- How much
- How long

The steps in Nursing Care Planning are:

- Determine priorities from the list of nursing diagnoses.
- Set long-term and short-term goals to determine outcomes of care.
- Develop objectives to reach the goals.
- Write nursing orders to direct care to meet the goals.

Measurement Criteria:

- The plan is individualized to the client's condition.
- The plan is developed with the client and significant others if appropriate.
- The plan reflects current nursing practice.
- The plan is documented.
- The plan provides for continuity of care.

IMPLEMENTATION

Implementation is the actual performance of the nursing interventions identified in the care plan. The implementations are coordinated with other members of the health care team who have direct care of the client. These interventions include, but are not limited to; health teaching, direct client care, medical treatments, medications, and dressing changes. Nurses provide care to achieve established goals of care and then communicate the nursing interventions by documenting and reporting. Not all interventions are planned. The nurse must use her critical thinking skills to respond to an unexpected crisis.

Measurement Criteria:

- Interventions are consistent with the established plan of care.
- Interventions are implemented in a safe and appropriate manner.
- Interventions are documented according to Nursing Standards.

The fourth step in the nursing process is implementation; Implementation involves the execution of the nursing, plan of care derived during the planning phase. It, comprises of performing nursing activities that have been, planned to meet the goals set with the client. Nurses, may delegate some of the nursing interventions to other, persons assigned to care for the client-for instance, the licensed practical nurses and unlicensed assistive, personnel., Implementation involves many skills. The nurse must, continue to evaluate the client's condition before, during, and after the nursing intervention.

Assessment prior to, the intervention provides the nurse with baseline data, Assessment during and after the intervention allows the, nurse to detect positive or negative responses the client, may have to the intervention. If negative responses, occur during the procedure, the nurse must take appropriate, action. If positive responses occur, the nurse adds, this information to the database for use in assessing, the efficacy of the intervention.

Five Activities of the Implementing Phase

- Ongoing evaluation: The nursing plan of care is based on the initial evaluation, data collected by the nurse and the nursing, diagnoses derived from those data. Because a client's, condition can change rapidly, or new data may become, available through interaction with the client, ongoing, evaluation is necessary to validate the relevance of proposed, interventions. Goals, expected outcomes, and, interventions may need to be altered as new data are, collected or progress toward outcomes is evaluated., Though a focused evaluation should be completed, during the initial interaction with the client, continuous, observations during the implementation process allow for adaptations to be made to better individualize care.
- Establishment of priorities: Following ongoing evaluation and review of the problem, list, and priorities are determined for implementation, of care. Priorities are based on: Which problems are viewed as most significant by the, nurse, the client, and family or significant others, Activities previously scheduled by other departments, (e.g., surgery, diagnostic testing), Available resources.
- Allocation of resources: Before implementing the nursing plan of care, the, nurse reviews proposed interventions to determine the, level of knowledge and the types of skills needed for, safe and effective implementation. The evaluation provides data for determining if an activity can be performed independently by the client, can be completed, with assistance from family, or requires assistance of, health care personnel.
- Initiation of nursing interventions: After reviewing the client's current condition, verifying priorities, and examining resources, the nurse should be ready, to initiate nursing interventions. A nursing intervention is, an action performed by the nurse that help the client to, achieve the results specified by the goals and expected outcomes. All interventions must conform to standards of care. Nurses should realize the reason for any intervention, the expected effect, and any potential problems that may, result. Understanding the reason for a nursing intervention, is the hallmark of a professional nurse, in that the nurse is, using logic and/or scientific reasoning as the basis of practice., Nursing interventions are a blend of science (rational, acts) and art (intuitive actions). It is significant for novice,

nurses to identify the rationale (the fundamental principle), of all interventions in order to implement theory-based practice.

- Documentation of interventions and client response: Communication concerning implementation of interventions, must be provided through written documentation, and should also be verbally conveyed when duty, of the client's care is transferred to another nurse., The nurse is legally needed to record all interventions and observations related to the client's response to treatment., This not only provides a legal record but also allows, valuable communication with other health care team, members for continuity of care and for assessing, progress toward expected outcomes. In addition, written, documentation provides data necessary for reimbursement, for services and tracking of indicators for continuous, quality improvement.

EVALUATION

Evaluation is an ongoing process that enables the nurse to determine what progress the patient has made in meeting the goals for care. The outcome criteria provide measures for determining outcomes of care.

In evaluating outcomes of care, determine whether goals have been met, partially met, or not met at all. If the goals have not been met it will be necessary to re-evaluate the plan. The plan may need to be altered, to do this you will need to do a new evaluation.

REFERENCES

Alfaro-LeFevre, R. (1998). Critical thinking in nursing: A practical approach (2nd ed.). Philadelphia: Saunders.

Beyer, B. K. (1987). Practical strategies for the teaching of thinking. Boston: Allyn & Bacon.

Bowman, S. (1999). Decision making and judgment for healthcare professionals. New York: Butterworth-Heinemann.

Brookfield, S. D. (1991). Developing critical thinkers. San Francisco: Jossey Bass.

Carpenito, L. J. (1999). Nursing diagnosis: Application to clinical practice (7th ed.). Philadelphia: Lippincott.

Edelman, C. L., & Mandle, C. L. (1997). Health promotion throughout the life span (4th ed.). St. Louis: Mosby.

Ennis, R. (1985). A logical basis for measuring critical thinking skills. Educational Leadership, 43(2), 44–48.

Fry, V. S. (1953). The creative approach to nursing. American Journal of Nursing, 53(3), 301–302.

Gebbie, K. M., & Lavin, M. A. (1974). Classifying nursing diagnoses. American Journal of Nursing, 74, 250–253.

Gilmartin, M. J. (1999). Creativity: The fuel of innovation. Nursing Administration Quarterly, 23(2), 1–8.

Jenkins, P., & Turick-Gibson, T. (1999). An exercise in critical thinking using role playing. Nurse Educator, 24(6), 11–14.

Johnson, D. (1959). A philosophy for nursing diagnosis. Nursing Outlook, 7, 198–200.

6

Documentation

Documentation is any written or electronically generated information about a client that describes the care or service provided to that client. Health records may be paper documents or electronic documents, such as electronic medical records, faxes, e-mails, audio or video tapes and images. Through documentation, nurses communicate their observations, decisions, actions and outcomes of these actions for clients. Documentation is an accurate account of what occurred and when it occurred. Nurses may document information pertaining to individual clients or groups of clients.

PURPOSE OF RECORDING AND REPORTING

To facilitate communication: Through documentation, nurses communicate to other nurses and care providers their evaluations about the status of clients, nursing interventions that are carried out and the results of these interventions. Documentation of this information increases the likelihood that the client will receive consistent and informed care or service. Thorough, accurate documentation decreases the potential for miscommunication and mistakes. While documentation is most often done by nurses and care providers, there are situations where the client and family may document observations or care provided in order to communicate this information with members of the health care team.

To promote good nursing care: Documentation encourages nurses to evaluate client progress and determine which interventions are effective and which are ineffective, and identify and document changes to the plan of care as required. Documentation can be a valuable source of data for making decisions about funding and resource management as well as facilitating nursing research, all of which have the potential to improve the quality of nursing practice and client care. Individual nurses can use outcome information or information from a critical incident to reflect on their practice and make required changes based on evidence.

To meet professional and legal standards: Documentation is a valuable method for demonstrating that, within the nurse-client relationship, the nurse has applied nursing knowledge, skills and judgment according to professional standards. The nurse's documentation may be used as evidence in legal proceedings such as lawsuits, coroners' inquests, and disciplinary hearings through professional regulatory bodies. In a court of law, the client's health record serves as the legal record of the care or service provided. Nursing care and the documentation of that care will be measured according to the standard of a reasonable and prudent nurse with similar education and experience in a similar situation.

COMMUNICATION WITHIN THE HEALTH CARE TEAM

Primary health care team members need to communicate effectively with each other in order to provide integrated care. Current theories about team working suggest that teams will be most effective if all members engage actively in discussion to set the team's goal and methods. Active discussion improves the degree to which persons realize the wider picture in the organization. The more explicit and agreed the group's goals, the better a group's performance when measured against those goals. Ideally, team working involves joint duty for decision-making, since this makes people more open and committed than they are in hierarchical structures. But even in groups where decision-making is centralized, communication is still significant to disseminate information about goals and plans to the group as a whole, and discussion to clarify these points is inevitable.

There are three pitfalls which could adversely affect primary care team discussions. The first is that the current business model for primary health care accentuates the status differences inherent in mixing staff with different amounts of clinical training. In most cases, doctors own their practices in partnership, employing most of the other staff. Status characteristics theory has shown that in mixed status groups, the higher status persons control discussions. In hierarchically organized workplaces, information flows down from the top but not up from the bottom, although this second direction of flow is essential for adapting working practice to a changing situation.

The second is the fact that some staff are employed directly by the practice, but other team members (most often, health visitors and district nurses), though attached to a specific practice or practices, report to outside agencies. Communication across such a divide is difficult, especially since the work of attached staff often takes them away from the practice premises. However, since goals across the divide will naturally differ to reflect the needs of the staff members' employers, this is where communication is most required.

The third is the common misconception that the best way to involve all staff members in setting group goals is to hold meetings to which everyone is invited. Large meetings are antithetical to coherent discussion. The more competition for the floor, the harder it is to say the right thing at the right time. They are also difficult to schedule, but in a conflict the disciplines with the least voice in the team are the most likely to be left out. Opportunities for informal communication can actually be just as significant, but because they are informal, they are not as often componented into group process design. Primary health care team practices which members might consider to be administrative details hence potentially have significant ramifications for patient care. In this study, we characterize the group communication processes of primary care teams, explore the relationship between communicative practice and team effectiveness, and discuss mechanisms for supporting the communication which these teams need.

TYPES OF RECORDS

When patients are in hospital or sick at home and visited by a nurse, it is important that the care they receive is recorded properly. Nurses record a wide variety of information about a patient's care and progress. For example, nurses would record a patient's status while in ICU every hour or when and how pain medication should be given and when it was given, or the progress of a pregnant woman visiting a clinic. These nursing records are a way for nurses to share care information with other nurses, other health care professionals and sometimes with patients. This is Information that can ensure patient care is consistent when staff changes shifts or information that can be used later as a history of previous care.

WARD RECORDS

A systematic review of the effect of nursing record systems on nursing practice found no evidence of effects on practice attributable to changes in record systems. Though there was a paucity of studies of sufficient methodological rigour for a Cochrane review, to yield reliable results in this area, it is clear from the literature that it is possible to set up randomised trials or other quasi-experimental designs required to produce evidence for practice. The review identified a need for research into the relationship between clinical practice and its understanding and written expression by nurses.

Effective nursing record systems may be as diverse as nursing practice itself. One study of unstructured record keeping ('scraps') suggested that the personal records kept in uniform pockets formed a significant part of the dynamic record of care, and that the structured formal documentation needs to be related to these scraps, and also the handover process. The challenge for nursing is to realize what characteristics of nursing practice are best served by which characteristics of record systems. For instance, which kind of practice needs a structured record, which kind needs to allow mostly free text? What aspects of nursing care need to be recorded and shared electronically, and which aspects of care are best served by a paper or voice format? A study on medical records systems suggested that the paper and electronic record are complementary for medical records. How will an effective nursing record be recognised? The latter is a fundamental question that cannot be answered until the intentions of record keeping have been fully articulated.

NURSING RECORDS

The nursing record forms part of the overall medical record for a patient and provides a formal record of the interaction between the nurse and the patient. It is also a form of communication between the nurse and other health professionals.

Nurses may record some details about patients other than in the nursing record, such as in informal notes. Still other observations may never be written down, especially behavioural, social, or psychological knowledge of the patient that often exists as tacit knowledge. Such tacit knowledge provides a richer context for understanding and treating the patient.

Traditionally, nursing records have been written on paper and kept in folders. These folders are typically divided into useful sections, with new information added to each section chronologically as the patient experiences new medical issues. Active records are usually housed at the clinical site, but older records (e.g., those of the deceased) are often kept in separate facilities.

The advent of electronic medical records has not only changed the format of nursing records but has increased accessibility of files. The use of an individual dossier style nursing record, where records are kept on each patient by name and illness type originated at the Mayo Clinic out of a desire to simplify patient tracking and to allow for medical research.

Although the specific content of the nursing record may vary depending upon specialty and location, it usually contains the patient's identification information, the patient's health history (what the patient tells the health-care providers about his or her past and present health status), and the patient's medical examination findings (what the health-care providers observe when the patient is examined). Other information may include lab test results; medications prescribed; referrals ordered to health-care providers; educational materials provided; and what plans there are for further care, including patient instruction for self-care and return visits. In some places, billing information is considered to be part of the nursing record.

Medical History

The medical history is a longitudinal record of what has happened to the patient since birth. It chronicles diseases, major and minor illnesses, as well as growth landmarks. It gives the clinician a feel for what has happened before to the patient. As a result, it may often give clues to current disease states. It includes several subsets detailed below.

Surgical history: The surgical history is a chronicle of surgery performed for the patient. It may have dates of operations, operative reports, and/or the detailed narrative of what the surgeon did.

Obstetric history: The obstetric history lists prior pregnancies and their outcomes. It also includes any complications of these pregnancies.

Medications and medical allergies: The medical record may contain a summary of the patient's current and previous medications as well as any medical allergies.

Family history: The family history lists the health status of immediate family members as well as their causes of death (if known). It may also list diseases common in the family or found only in one sex or the other. It may also include a pedigree chart. It is a valuable asset in predicting some outcomes for the patient.

Social history: The social history is a chronicle of human interactions. It tells of the relationships of the patient, his/her careers and trainings, schooling and religious training. It is helpful for the physician to know what sorts of community support the patient might expect during a major illness. It may explain the behaviour of the patient in relation to illness or loss. It may also give clues as to the cause of an illness (e.g. occupational exposure to asbestos).

Habits: Various habits which impact health, such as tobacco use, alcohol intake, recreational drug use, exercise, and diet are chronicled, often as part of the social history. This section may also include more intimate details such as sexual habits and sexual preferences.

Immunization history: The history of vaccination is included. Any blood tests proving immunity will also be included in this section.

Growth chart and developmental history: For children and teenagers, charts documenting growth as it compares to other children of the same age is included, so that health-care providers can follow the child's growth over time. Many diseases and social stresses can affect growth and longitudinal charting and can thus provide a clue to underlying illness. Additionally, a child's behaviour (such as timing of talking, walking, etc.) as it compares to other children of the same age is documented within the medical record for much the same reasons as growth.

Progress Notes

When a patient is hospitalized, daily updates are entered into the medical record documenting clinical changes, new information, etc. These often take the form of a SOAP note and are entered by all members of the health-care team (doctors, nurses, physical therapists, dieticians, clinical pharmacists, respiratory therapists, etc). They are kept in chronological order and document the sequence of events leading to the current state of health.

Test Results

The results of testing, such as blood tests (e.g., complete blood count) radiology examinations (e.g., X-rays), pathology (e.g., biopsy results), or specialized testing (e.g., pulmonary function testing) are included. Often, as in the case of X-rays, a written report of the findings is included in lieu of the actual film.

Other Information

Many other items are variably kept within the medical record. Digital images of the patient, flow sheets from operations/intensive care units, informed consent forms, EKG tracings, outputs from medical devices (such as pacemakers), chaemotherapy protocols, and numerous other important pieces of information form part of the record depending on the patient and his or her set of illnesses/treatments.

There is various information needed to be recorded while tracing state of patient's daily health:

1. Vital Signs: Body Temperature, Pulse Rate (Heart Rate), Blood Pressure and Respiratory Rate.
2. Intake: Medication, Fluid, Nutrition, Water and Blood, etc.
3. Output: Blood, Urine, Excrement, Vomitus and Sweat, etc.
4. Observation on Pupil size.
5. Capability of four limbs of body

COMMON RECORD KEEPING FORMS

Various types of forms in use in the hospital can be classified under the following broad categories;

- Forms used for patient care activities
- Forms used for administrative intentions

FORMS FOR PATIENT CARE

Records kept by Doctors:

- Face Sheet
- Discharge Summary
- General History & Physical Examination
- Progress Record
- Doctor's Orders
- Consultation Record
- Operation Record
- Anaesthesia Record

Records kept by nurses:

- Intake Output Chart
- Temperature, Pulse, Respiration Chart
- Nurses Daily Record
- Consent Form

Diagnostic forms:

- Laboratory Forms, including Haematology, Microbiology, Clinical Chemistry
- Tissue report forms (Histopathology)
- Other investigation report forms e.g., X-ray, ECG etc.

- Special Investigation Report Forms e.g., Radio isotope studies, MRI, Pulmonary Function test, Clinical Immunology. Hormone assay, Bone densitometry request forms etc.

Department specific forms:

- For outpatients - Specialty Clinic Proforma, e.g., Diabetes Clinic proforma in Endocrinology, Liver Clinic Proforma in Gastroenterology etc.
- For inpatients - Special forms for NICU, Nephrology, Orthopaedics, Urology, Paediatric Surgery etc.

FORMS FOR ADMINISTRATIVE PURPOSES

- Admission slip
- Medical & Fitness Certificate
- Reimbursement forms
- Estimates

COMPUTERISED DOCUMENTATION

A client's electronic health record is a collection of the personal health information of a single individual, entered or accepted by health care providers, and stored electronically, under strict security. As with traditional or paper-based systems, documentation in electronic health records must be comprehensive, accurate, timely, and clearly identify who provided what care. Entries are made by the provider providing the care and not by other staff. Entries made and stored in an electronic health record are considered a permanent part of the record and may not be deleted. If corrections are needed to the entry after the entry has been stored, agency policies provide direction as to how this should occur. Most agencies using electronic documentation have policies to support its use, including policies for:

- Correcting documentation mistakes or making "late entries";
- Preventing the deletion of information;
- Identifying changes and updates to the record;
- Protecting the confidentiality of client information;
- Maintaining the security of the system (passwords, virus protection, encryption, firewalls);
- Tracking unauthorized access to client information;
- Processes for documenting in agencies using a mix of electronic and paper methods;

- Backing-up client information; and
- Means of documentation in the event of a system failure.

The use of e-mail by health care organizations and health care professionals is becoming more widespread as a result of its speed, reliability, convenience and low cost. Unfortunately the components that make the use of e-mail so advantageous also pose significant confidentiality, security and legal risks. E-mail can be likened to sending a postcard. It is not sealed, and may be read by anyone. Because the security and confidentiality of e-mail cannot be guaranteed, it is not recommended as a method for transmission of health information. Messages can easily be misdirected to or intercepted by an unintended recipient. The information can then be read, forwarded and/or printed. Though messages on a local computer can be deleted, they are never deleted from the central server routing the message and can, in fact, be retrieved. Having considered these risks and alternative ways to transmit health information, e-mail may be the preferred option to meet client needs in some cases.

From the nurse's perspective, it is significant to realize that e-mail messages are a form of client documentation and are stored electronically or printed in hard copy and placed in the client's health record. E-mails are part of the client's permanent record and, if relevant, can be subject to disclosure in legal proceedings. E-mail messages are written with this in mind. Similar to physicians' orders received by fax, if physicians' orders are received by e-mail, nurses use whatever means necessary to confirm the authenticity of the orders.

Guidelines for Using Electronic Health Records

Guidelines for nurses using electronic health records are as follows:

- Never reveal or allow anyone else access to your personal identification number or password as these are, in
- Fact, electronic signatures;
- Inform your immediate supervisor if there is suspicion that an assigned personal identification code is being
- Used by someone else;
- Change passwords at frequent and irregular intervals (as per agency policy);
- Choose passwords that are not easily deciphered;
- Log off when not using the system or when leaving the terminal;

- Maintain confidentiality of all information, including all print copies of information;
- Shred any discarded print information containing client identification;
- Locate printers in secured areas away from public access;
- Retrieve printed information immediately;
- Protect client information displayed on monitors (e.g., use of screen saver, location of monitor, use of privacy screens);
- Use only systems with secured access to record client information;
- Only access client information which is needed to provide nursing care for that client; accessing client information for intentions other than providing nursing care is a breach of confidentiality.

GUIDELINES FOR REPORTING

Reporting is the verbal communication of data regarding the client's health status, needs, treatments, outcomes, and responses. When a report is given, it needs to summarize the current critical information that facilitates clinical decision making and continuity of care. As with recording, reporting is based on the nursing process, standards of care, and legal and ethical principles. The nursing process provides structure for an organized report, a challenge inherent in verbal communications. In order to verbally communicate an efficient and well-organized report, the nurse must consider:

- What needs to be said
- Why it needs to be said
- How to say it
- What the expected outcomes are

Considering these aspects of reporting before the communication will provide for a concise, organized report. Another critical element in reporting is listening. Reports require participation from everyone present. When receiving a report, the nurse focuses behaviours to enhance listening skills: the nurse eliminates distractions, puts thoughts and concerns aside, concentrates on what is being said, and does not anticipate what the presenter will say next. The reporting process is an integral component of developing effective interpersonal and intrapersonal relationships that promote continuity of client care. Regardless of the type of communication, planned presentation of client data is a key to accurate, concise, effective reporting. Summary reports, walking rounds, telephone reports and orders, and incident reports are all types of reporting.

SUMMARY REPORTS

Summary reports summarize pertinent client information that focuses on the client's needs as identified by the nursing process for the new caregiver. Summary reports commonly occur at the change of shift and when the client is transferred to another area. A summary, or end-of-shift, report should be presented as follows:

- Background data obtained from client interactions and assessment of the functional health patterns
- Primary medical and nursing diagnoses and priority problems
- Identification of client risk problems
- Recent changes in condition or in treatments (e.g., new medications, elevated temperature)
- Effective interventions or treatments of priority problems, inclusive of laboratory and diagnostic results (e.g., client's response to pain medication)
- Progress toward expected outcomes: priority problems, teaching or discharge planning
- Adjustments in the plan of care
- Client or family complaints

This format will provide structure and organization to the data that are both logical and time-sequenced since the format follows the nursing process. The new caregiver needs to receive an accurate, concise report about what has happened during the previous shift in order to provide continuity of care. Client and family complaints should be addressed last for each client because these situations usually generate questions and discussion.

METHODS OF RECORDING

Most methods of documentation fall into one of two categories: documentation by inclusion and documentation by exception. Documentation by inclusion is done on an ongoing, regular basis and makes note of all evaluation findings, nursing interventions and client outcomes. Documentation by exception, on the other hand, makes note of negative findings and is completed when evaluation findings, nursin interventions or client outcomes vary from the established evaluatio norms or standards of care existing within a particular agency. Chartin by exception replaces the long held belief of "if it was not charted, then i was not done" with a new premise, "all standards have been met with normal or expected response unless documented otherwise."

1. Documentation by exception is only appropriate when evaluatio norms or standards of care are explicitly written and availabl within the agency. Documentation by exception is neve acceptable for medication administration.
2. The documentation method selected within an agency or practic setting needs to reflect client care needs and the context o practice. Some agencies may combine elements of differen documentation methods and formats. If an agency decides t change its method or format of documentation and/o expectations, it is significant that this be done within a contex of appropriate planning and includes the involvement an education of nurses.
3. Regardless of the method used, nurses are accountable an responsible for documenting client evaluations, intervention carried out, and the impact of the interventions on clien outcomes. Clients who are very ill, considered high risk, o have complex health problems generally require mor comprehensive, in-depth and frequent documentation.
4. Three common documentation methods - focus charting SOAP/SOAPIER and narrative documentation are described i the following sections. Any of these methods may be used t document on an inclusion or exception basis.

FOCUS CHARTING

With this method of documentation, the nurse identifies a "focus" based on client concerns or behaviours determined during the evaluation For instance, a focus could reflect:

- A current client concern or behaviour, such as decrease urinary output.
- A change in a client's condition or behaviour, such a disorientation to time, place and individual.
- A significant event in the client's treatment, such as retur from surgery.

- In focus charting, the evaluation of client status, the interventions carried out and the impact of the interventions on client outcomes are organized under the headings of data, action and response.
- Data: Subjective and/or objective information that supports the stated focus or describes the client status at the time of a significant event or intervention.
- Action: Completed or planned nursing interventions based on the nurse's evaluation of the client's status.
- Response: Description of the impact of the interventions on client outcomes.

Flow sheets and checklists are frequently used as an adjunct to document routine and ongoing evaluations and observations such as personal care, vital signs, intake and output, etc. Information recorded on flow sheets or checklists does not need to be repeated in the progress notes.

SOAP CHARTING

The SOAP note (an acronym for subjective, objective, assessment, and plan) is a method of documentation employed by doctors and other health care providers to write out notes in a patient's chart, along with other common formats, such as the admission note. Documenting patient encounters in the medical record is an integral part of practice workflow starting with patient appointment scheduling, to writing out notes, to medical billing. Prehospital care providers such as EMTs may use the same format to communicate patient information to Emergency department clinicians.

Components

The four components of a SOAP note are Subjective, Objective, Assessment, and Plan. The length and focus of each component of a SOAP note varies depending on the specialty; for instance, a surgical SOAP note is likely to be much briefer than a medical SOAP note, and will focus on issues that relate to post-surgical status.

Subjective component: This describes the patient's current condition in narrative form. The history or state of experienced symptoms are recorded in the patient's own words. It will include all pertinent and negative symptoms under review of body systems. Pertinent Medical history, surgical history, family history, social history along with current medications and allergies are also recorded. A SAMPLE history is one method of obtaining this information from a patient.

If this is the first time a doctor is seeing a patient, they will take a History of Present Illness or HPI. To structure this portion of the note, you can use another mnemonic: OLD CHARTS, as in what would you find if you looked at the patient's "old chart"

- Onset
- Location
- Duration
- CHaracter (sharp, dull, etc)
- Alleviating/Aggravating factors
- Radiation
- Temporal pattern (every morning, all day, etc)
- Symptoms associated

Objective component: The objective component includes:

- Vital signs
- Findings from physical examinations, such as posture, bruising, and abnormalities
- Results from laboratory tests
- Measurements, such as age and weight of the patient.

Assessment: Is a quick summary of the patient with main symptoms/ diagnosis including a differential diagnosis, a list of other possible diagnoses usually in order of most likely to least likely. When used in a Problem Oriented Medical Record, relevant problem numbers or headings are included as subheadings in the assessment.

Plan: This is what the health care provider will do to treat the patient's concerns. This should address each item of the differential diagnosis. A note of what was discussed or advised with the patient as well as timings for further review or follow-up may also be included.

NARRATIVE CHARTING

Narrative charting is a method in which nursing interventions and the impact of these interventions on client outcomes are recorded in chronological order covering a specific time frame. Data is recorded in the progress notes, often without an organizing framework. Narrative charting may stand alone or it may be complemented by other tools, such as flow sheets and checklists.

USE OF TECHNOLOGY

Technology may be used to support client documentation in a number of ways. If technology is used, the principles underlying documentation, access, storage, retrieval and transmittal of information remain the same as for a traditional, paper-based system. These new ways of recording, delivering and receiving client information, nevertheless, pose significant challenges for nurses, particularly with respect to confidentiality and security of client information. It is significant that nurses be supported by agencies in resolving these issues through clear policies and rules and ongoing education.

REPORTING

WALKING ROUNDS

Walking rounds can be either nursing rounds, physician nurse rounds, or interdisciplinary rounds. Walking rounds is a reporting method used when the members of the care team walk to each client's room and discuss care and progress with each other and with the client. Nursing rounds are used most frequently by charge nurses as their method of report. During the rounds, the on-coming nurse is introduced to the client and the off-going nurse discusses with the client and the oncoming nurse changes in the plan of care. Rounds are more time-consuming than the end-of-shift report but give the nurses and the client the opportunity to evaluate the effectiveness of care together. Nursing rounds are also used as a teaching method. The instructor introduces the client to the student, and together they discuss the client's care. The instructor can also use this time to appraise the student's observation, communication, and decision-making skills.

Nurse-physician rounds can involve either the staff nurse or the charge nurse with the physician.

These rounds usually occur daily and provide the nurse, physician, and client the opportunity to evaluate the effectiveness of care. Interdisciplinary rounds, in which many disciplines are involved, usually occur less frequently than the other types of rounds. Continuity of care, patient satisfaction, and decreased costs are often the outcomes of daily interdisciplinary rounds. The interdisciplinary concept recognizes that health care providers do not work independently of one another, but address patients' needs within the context of all team members. Interdisciplinary rounds are done most commonly in place of or to supplement case conferences and to discuss discharge planning.

Interdisciplinary rounds support the concept of critical pathways and are seen most frequently in teaching hospitals.

CHANGE-OF SHIFT REPORTS

At the end of a long day of caring for patients, it's time to give the end-of-shift report to the oncoming nurses. Though it may be tempting to rush through this routine duty, patient safety hinges on a complete and correct exchange of information.

One of the most frequent mistakes during a shift report is inadvertently omitting critical safety information.

There are three key safety areas to cover: allergies, code status and medical team members. Allergy information is critical, because it may dictate which medications can be safely administered to a patient. Code status includes information about whether a patient wants to be resuscitated. Finally, oncoming nurses need to know the members of the patient's medical team in case a nurse needs to call for help.

In addition to safety information, an outgoing nurse must inform the oncoming nurse about a patient's medical history and current condition. This information needs to be conveyed methodically, such as moving through each body system (cardiac, urinary, etc.) or going from head to toe.

Another key piece of information is the patient's future care plan. The future care plan is one of the most significant things that can be missed. A nurse should always know where she is heading, because this prioritizes what she is doing.

For instance, a nurse who is ending a shift may know that a patient will be going to the operating room for a procedure. The oncoming nurse needs to know this so she can be sure the patient does not eat.

TELEPHONE REPORTS AND ORDERS

Telephone communications are another way nurses report transfers, communicate referrals, obtain client data, solve problems, and inform a physician and/or client's family members regarding a change in the client's condition. Nurses are expected to demonstrate phone courtesy and professionalism when initiating and receiving telephone reports and orders. When initiating a phone call, organize the information to be reported or received. For example:

1. Make sure all lab results are back; if they are not, identify in advance, which ones are missing and phone the lab or check

the computer to determine if other results are available. Write down which tests have been performed and the results. Spell the client's name and provide the client's medical record number to avoid error in getting the results on the wrong client.

2. Review your notes, have your assessment data readily available, especially any significant client data that are related to the call. If you have not assessed the client, do an assessment before telephoning the practitioner; otherwise, the practitioner might ask you questions that you will not be able to answer.

3. Let the charge nurse or someone else at the nurses' station know that you are placing the call so that you will not be interrupted while on the phone. When you place the call, state the reason you are calling: for example, "I am calling Dr. Sharma regarding the blood sugar results for Mrs. Asha Gupta." Be brief and listen carefully. Repeat the test results and any orders the physician gives over the phone.

Record accurately in the medical record the date and time the phone call was placed, the client data you reported on the phone, the name of the person you spoke with, and whether an order was obtained. Do not chart "physician notified, no orders obtained." Rather, chart "Dr. Sharma notified by phone, blood sugar 260 mg (drawn by the lab at 1300), orders received and recorded on the physician order sheet." Charting telephone orders and documentation in the nurses' progress notes should be done as soon as possible after the phone call to prevent an entry by another caregiver before you chart the telephone report.

Record the order as given by the physician; then sign the order beginning with t.o. (telephone order), write the physician's name, and sign your name. If another nurse witnesses the phone order, that nurse's signature should go after yours. The physician needs to countersign the order within a time frame as specified by the facility's policy. Fax machines have decreased the need for lengthy or complicated telephone orders, both saving time and avoiding error. To confirm the physician's identity as the initiator of the fax orders, telephone the physician. The physician needs to countersign the fax orders according to agency policy.

INCIDENT REPORTS

Incident reports, or occurrence reports, are used to document any unusual occurrence or accident in the delivery of client care, such as falls or medication errors. The Code for Nurses states that nurses are expected "to protect the client when safety is affected." Ethical practice requires that nurses file an incident report to protect the client not to punish the caregiver.

The filing of incident reports is not only an internal device for the facility but is also a requirement by federal, national, and state accrediting agencies. Nurses are often advised not to document the filing of an incident report in the nurses' notes for legal reasons, but, as previously discussed, documenting medication errors requires an incident report and documentation in the nurses' notes to ensure that the client receives safe care. The incident report serves two functions:

1. It informs the facility's administration of the incident, so risk management personnel can consider changes that might prevent similar occurrences in the future.
2. It alerts the facility's insurance company to a potential claim and the need for further investigation. Litigation can be avoided if the facility takes prompt action by investigating an occurrence. The incident report is not part of the medical record, but it may be used later in litigation. Each person with firsthand knowledge of the occurrence should fill out and sign a separate report. Although the incident report format varies from one facility to another, there are key elements that must be addressed when filing a report:

- Record the date, exact time, and place you discovered the occurrence.
- Identify the person(s) involved in the occurrence, including witnesses.
- Document accurately and objectively the exact occurrences that you witnessed or first saw after the incident; for example, record "found the client sitting on the floor. Client stated that..." rather than "client fell."
- Record the exact details, in time sequence, what happened, and the consequences for the persons involved.
- Record your actions to provide care and results of your assessment for injuries or client complaints.
- Notify the supervisor on duty and record the time and name of the physician notified; if telephone orders were received from the physician, document as previously discussed and implement the orders.

- Do not record your opinions, judgments, conclusions, or assumptions about what occurred, point blame, or suggest how to prevent occurrence of a similar incident.
- Forward the incident report to the designated person as defined in the facility's policy.

MINIMIZING LEGAL LIABILITY THROUGH EFFECTIVE RECORD KEEPING

Most nurses dislike paperwork - especially which involved in entering information in medical records. This often means that entering data into the medical chart is delegated to a junior or inexperienced assistant, as a result of which it is often not done well.

Remember that the medical record serves many intentions, and its primary function is to plan for patient care. However, from the risk management perspective, the nursing record is a crucial element in preventing and minimizing malpractice litigation. Ultimately, it serves as the basis for the defence of malpractice claims and lawsuits. Nursing records which are poorly maintained, incomplete, inaccurate, illegible or altered, create doubt about the treatment given to a patient, and can be a major medical-legal liability. By contrast, proper documentation in the nursing record creates a legal document which accurately and completely reflects the care provided to a patient and, in a courtroom setting, it may be likened to a witness whose memory is never lost.

While keeping good records is simply a matter of common sense, the mnemonic OLFACTORY, which stands for: Original, Legible, Factual, Accurate, Complete, Timely, Objective, Rationale and Yours, will help you to define a "good" nursing record.

It is helpful to follow a system when making notes in the nursing record, to ensure that all significant information has been recorded. The SOAP system [which stands for Subjective (the patient's history); Objective (examination findings); Assessment and Plan] is popular in many hospitals, and is easy to implement. Pre-printed nursing records can help to establish consistent documentation, ensuring you do not forget to record significant information. They can also help to save your time when entering data.

When writing orders in the chart, it can be helpful to remember the following headings (ADCA VAN DIMS), to ensure that significant orders are not overlooked. Every nurse should develop their own systematic method to ensure completeness.

- Admission
- Diagnosis
- Condition
- Allergies
- Vital signs
- Ambulation
- Nursing care
- Diet
- IV fluids
- Lab tests
- Medications
- Special orders (such as occupational therapy or consultations requested)

Each and every page of a patient record should be clearly labelled with the patient's complete name and nursing record number. Anyone making an entry in a patient's chart should do so only on hospital approved nursing record forms and then only with pen rather than pencil. Use only hospital accepted medical abbreviations and terminology. Associated records and tests such as EKG's, EEG's, foetal monitoring tracings, etc., should all be correctly labelled with the patient's name, medical record number, the date and time.

REFERENCES

Ackley, B. J., & Ladwig, G. B. (1997). Nursing diagnostic handbook (3rd ed.). St. Louis: Mosby Year-Book.

Andrews, H., & Roy, C. (1991). The Roy Adaptation Model: The definitive statement. Norwalk, CT: Appleton & Lange.

Doenges, M. E., & Moorhouse, M. F. (1995). Application of nursing process and nursing diagnosis (2nd ed.). Philadelphia: F. A. Davis.

Estes, M. Z. (1998). Health assessment and physical examination. Albany, NY: Delmar Publishers.

Gordon, M. (1997). Manual of nursing diagnoses 1997–1998 edition. St. Louis: Mosby.

Norwood, B. R. (1997). The nursing process. In K. K. Chitty, (Ed.), Professional nursing: Concepts and challenges (2nd ed.). Philadelphia: W. B. Saunders.

Orem, D. E. (1995). Nursing: Concepts of practice. (5th ed.). St. Louis: Mosby.

Sparks, S. M., & Taylor, C. M. (1995). Nursing diagnosis reference manual (3rd ed.). Springhouse, PA: Springhouse.

Wilkinson, J. M. (1995). Nursing process: A critical thinking approach. Menlo Park, CA: Addison-Wesley.

7

Vital Signs

Patient observations are a significant part of nursing care in that they allow the patient's progress to be monitored and also ensure prompt detection of adverse events or delayed recovery. Patient observations, or vital signs, traditionally consist of blood pressure, temperature, pulse rate and respiratory rate. A systematic study was recently conducted addressing issues such as the intention of vital signs, the optimal frequency with which they should be conducted, what observations constitute vital signs and to identify issues related to the individual measures of temperature, pulse rate, respiratory rate and blood pressure.

The measurement of temperature, pulse, heart rate and blood pressure is termed both vital signs and observations. Neither have been well defined and their use is inconsistent and at times interchangeable. The term vital signs suggests measurement of vital or critical physiologic functions, where as the term "observations" implies broader range of measures. While there is no clear definition in the literature, a panel of experts argued that observations is the more appropriate term, in that it more accurately reflects current clinical practice. This implies that patient observations need not be limited to the traditional four parametres but supplemented with other measures as indicated by the patient's clinical status.

Traditionally, the term "vital signs" is used in reference to the measurement of temperature, respiratory rate, pulse rate and blood pressure. However, within the literature there are suggestions that these parametres could be supplemented with other useful measures such as nutritional status, smoking status, spirometry, orthostatic vital signs and pulse oximetry. However, only pulse oximetry and determining a patient's smoking status have been shown to actually change the practice of clinicians.

Studies have demonstrated that in some situations pulse oximetry is useful for detecting a deterioration in physiological function that might otherwise be missed. This has resulted in a reduction in the number of investigations undertaken and has changed the planned management of patients. On this basis, pulse oximetry has been recommended as a useful addition to the four traditional measures of physiologic status.

There is only limited information regarding the frequency with which patient observation should be undertaken and much of this is based on surveys of nurses, clinical practice reports and expert opinion. Surveys of nurses have shown that many admit to carrying out frequent vital sign measurements on patients they believed didn't require them, and that they had become a routine procedure unrelated to perceived individual patients needs.

GUIDELINES FOR TAKING VITAL SIGNS

As there may be no knowledge of the patient's previous vital signs for comparison, it is significant that the nurse be aware that there is a wide range of normal values that can apply to patients of different ages. The nurse should take as detailed a medical history from the patient as possible; any known medical or surgical history, prior measurements of vital signs, and details of current medication(s) should be recorded on the patient's chart. Any physical exertion prior to measurement of vital signs, such as climbing stairs, may affect the measurements. Thirty minutes prior to the taking of one's vital signs, the patient should not have consumed tobacco, caffeinated drinks, or alcohol.

Blood pressure is taken using a cuff that is the correct size for the patient; this will provide the most accurate reading. The reading can be 10 to 50 millimetres (mm) Hg too high with a cuff that is too small; a false reading of hypertension (high blood pressure) may result.

All types of sphygmomanometers-a cuff that can be filled with air, a hollow rubber bulb that pumps the air, and a glass tube that contains a column of mercury-should be calibrated annually by a trained technician. This will ensure that equipment remains accurate.

- Vital signs are recorded from once hourly to four times hourly, and as needed by the patient's condition.
- Temperature is recorded to check for pyrexia (a febrile condition) or to monitor the degree of hypothermia.
- The pulse is checked for any abnormalities of the heart by measuring the rate, rhythm, and regularity of the beat, as well as the strength and tension of the beat against the arterial wall.

- Blood pressure is recorded for older children and adults. A normal blood pressure reading is 120/70.

The patient should be made comfortable and reassured that recording vital signs is part of normal health checks, and that it is necessary to ensure that his or her health is being properly monitored. Any abnormalities in the vital signs must be reported to the medical staff.

The vital signs are recorded and compared with normal ranges for the patient's age and medical condition. Based on these results, it is decided whether any further action needs to be taken.

BODY TEMPERATURE

PHYSIOLOGY

Body temperature is the average temperature maintained within the body. It varies locally: extremities and tissue near the surface may be somewhat cooler. The average normal human body temperature is considered 36.5°Celsius, or 98.6°Fahrenheit. This varies slightly according to such components as the individual, the time of day, state of metabolism and physical activity, and temperature of surroundings. A high temperature is often a sign of fever; a low temperature may be a sign of hypothermia, death, or other anomalies.

FACTORS AFFECTING BODY TEMPERATURE

Body temperature can also be typically affected by such things as extreme physical activity, ovulation and pregnancy in women, and smoking. It is also affected by the part of the body measured: The body's extremities are colder than the body core; and temperature taken in the mouth, while convenient, tends to be less accurate (due to improper thermometer placement, breathing, recent consumption of hot or cold beverages, etc.) than temperature measured rectally or tympanically, but more accurate than axillary measurements. Strenuous exercise can temporarily raise body temperature to as high as 103°F, while extreme exercise, such as a marathon, can raise body temperature temporarily as high as 107°F.

ASSESSMENT OF BODY TEMPERATURE

Sites

A person's body temperature can be taken in any of the following ways:

- Orally: Temperature can be taken by mouth using either the classic glass thermometer, or the more modern digital thermometers that use an electronic probe to measure body temperature.
- Rectally: Temperatures taken rectally (using a glass or digital thermometer) tend to be 0.5 to 0.7° F higher than when taken by mouth.
- Axillary: Temperatures can be taken under the arm using a glass or digital thermometer. Temperatures taken by this route tend to be 0.3 to 0.4° F lower than those temperatures taken by mouth.
- By Ear: A special thermometer can quickly measure the temperature of the ear drum, which reflects the body's core temperature (the temperature of the internal organs).

Equipments

- Electronic thermometers are plastic and shaped like a pencil, with a display window at one end and the temperature probe at the other end. They work by measuring how well electricity travels through a wire. Electronic thermometers are used in the mouth, rectum, or armpit. They are easy to use, easy to read, and are accurate.
- Ear thermometers are plastic and come in different shapes. They use infrared energy to measure body temperature. The small cone-shaped end of the thermometer is placed in the ear, and body temperature shown on a digital display. The results appear within seconds.
- Forehead thermometers use skin temperature to determine body temperature. Some have a soft disc that are pressed against the forehead and show the temperature on a digital display. Other types are thin pieces of plastic with numbers on them. You press the strip against a person's forehead, and the temperature makes some numbers change colours or light up.
- Disposable thermometers are thin flat pieces of plastic with coloured dots and temperature markings on one end. The colour of the dots shows the temperature. Disposable thermometers can be used in the mouth or rectum. A patch form can be used on a baby's skin to measure temperature continuously for 48 hours. These thermometers are safe and accurate within

0.2°F (0.1°C). They do not contain glass, latex, or mercury.

- Pacifier thermometers are shaped like a baby's pacifier but have a display that shows the temperature. The pacifier thermometer is placed in child's mouth to measure temperature.

Technique

Oral is the most common method of taking a temperature. To get an accurate temperature, the individual must be able to breathe through the nose. If this is impossible because of a stuffy nose or lack of cooperation, use the rectum or armpit.

- The digital or disposable thermometer is placed under the tongue, just to one side of the centre, and lips are closed tightly around it.
- Leave the thermometer in place for the needed amount of time. Time with a clock or watch.
- Remove the thermometer and read it.
- Clean a digital thermometer with cool, soapy water and rinse it off before putting it away.

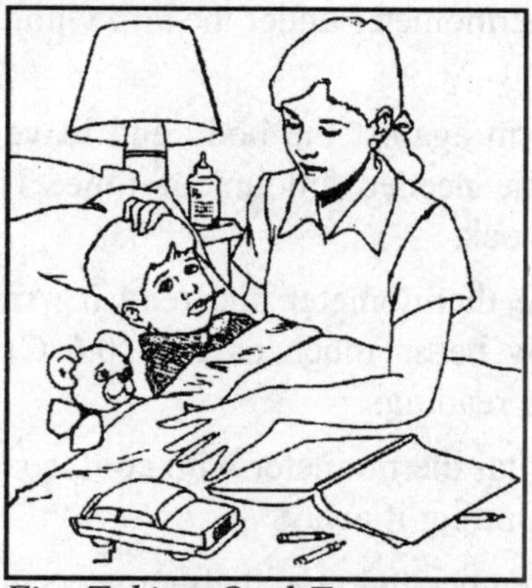

Fig. Taking Oral Temperature

Taking a Rectal Temperature: This is the location to measure body temperature most accurately. It is recommended for babies, small children, and people who cannot hold a thermometer safely in their mouths. It is also used when getting the most accurate measurement is essential.

- Apply a lubricant jelly or petroleum jelly, such as Vaseline, on the bulb of the thermometer so that you can insert it easily.
- When measuring the temperature of babies or small children, turn the child face down on the lap or on a flat covered or padded surface, such as a bed.

- Spread the child's buttocks with one hand and gently insert the bulb end of the rectal thermometer about 0.5 in. (1.25 cm) to 1 in. (2.5 cm) into the anal canal with your other hand. Don't force it into the rectum. Hold the thermometer in place with two fingers close to the anal opening (not near the end of the thermometer). Pressing the child's buttocks together will help keep the thermometer in place.
- Leave the thermometer in place for the needed amount of time.
- Remove the thermometer and read it. A rectal temperature reading may be as much as 1°F (0.6°C) higher than an oral temperature reading.
- Clean a digital thermometer with cool, soapy water and rinse it off before putting it away.
- Do not use a thermometer to take an oral temperature after it has been used to take a rectal temperature.

Taking an Armpit (axillary) Temperature: Taking a temperature in the armpit may not be as accurate as taking an oral or rectal temperature.

- Place the thermometer under the arm with the bulb in the centre of the armpit.
- Press the arm against the body and leave the thermometer in place for the needed amount of time. Time yourself with a watch or clock.
- Remove the thermometer and read it. An armpit temperature reading may be as much as 1°F (0.6°C) lower than an oral temperature reading.
- Clean a digital thermometer with cool, soapy water and rinse it off before putting it away.

Taking an Ear Temperature: Ear thermometers may need to be cleaned and prepared for use. These steps can be followed when using an ear thermometer.

- Check that the probe is clean and free of debris. If dirty, wipe it gently with a clean cloth. Do not immerse the thermometer in water.
- To keep the probe clean, a disposable probe cover should be used. Use a new probe cover each time you take an ear temperature. Attach the disposable cover to the probe.
- Turn the thermometer on.

- For babies younger than 12 months, pull the earlobe down and back. This will help place the probe in the ear canal. Centre the probe tip in the ear and push gently inward toward the eardrum.
- For children older than 12 months and for adults, pull the earlobe up and back. Centre the probe tip in the ear and push gently inward toward the eardrum.
- Press the "on" button to display the temperature reading.
- Remove the thermometer and throw away the used probe cover.

Taking a Forehead Temperature: Press the soft cup of the thermometer or the entire plastic strip firmly against a dry forehead. Hold the thermometer in place for the needed amount of time. Time yourself with a watch or clock.

Read the temperature before removing the thermometer. Clean the thermometer with cool soapy water and rinse it off before putting it away. Forehead thermometers are not as accurate as electronic and ear thermometers. If your baby is younger than 3 months or your child's fever rises higher than 102° (39°), recheck the temperature using a better method.

TEMPERATURE ALTERATIONS

Hyperthermia

Hyperthermia, in its advanced state referred to as heat stroke or sunstroke, is an acute condition which occurs when the body produces or absorbs more heat than it can dissipate. It is commonly caused by prolonged exposure to high temperatures. The heat-regulating mechanisms of the body eventually become overwhelmed and unable to effectively deal with the heat, causing the body temperature to climb uncontrollably. Hyperthermia is a medical emergency which requires immediate treatment.

Hypothermia

Hypothermia is a condition in which an organism's temperature drops below that needed for normal metabolism and bodily functions. In warm-blooded animals, core body temperature is maintained near a constant level through biologic homeostasis. But, when the body is exposed to cold, its internal mechanisms may be unable to replenish the heat that is being lost to the organism's surroundings. Hypothermia is the opposite of hyperthermia, the condition that causes heat exhaustion and heat stroke.

Heatstroke

Heat stroke is a form of hyperthermia, an abnormally elevated body temperature with accompanying physical and neurological symptoms. Unlike heat cramps and heat exhaustion, two forms of hyperthermia that are less severe, heat stroke is a true medical emergency that can be fatal if not correctly and promptly treated.

HOT AND COLD APPLICATIONS

With heat therapy, temperature alterations have four main effects on surface body tissues, including pain relief (analgesia), muscle relaxation, blood vessel alterations, and connective tissue effects. By reducing the speed of impulses conducted by nerve fibres, pain sensations are inhibited by cold. Target temperatures of 10-15°C are recommended. Similarly, decreases in muscle spasm are seen with cold therapy, though the exact mechanisms for this are unclear. It is thought that this result may be mediated through reflex reduction in motor nerve activity secondary to response to increased activity in cold receptors. With regard to the circulatory system, cold causes constriction of small arteries and veins, by direct stimulation of the smooth muscle lining these vessels. However, a curious reverse relaxing effect occurs with very low temperatures or prolonged cooling. The benefits of vasoconstriction include decreased haemorrhage and swelling within injured tissues, though some animal studies have shown a paradoxical increase in swelling with cold application.

The common therapeutic techniques include direct application of ice or snow, the use of special cold packs or compression devices (using ice water or cooled water; 10-25°C), cold water baths (hydrotherapy) or cooling topical sprays. These techniques utilize conduction and convection as means of cooling affected areas. General rules include the need to protect the skin from cold injury via a layer of intervening material, and limiting exposures to twenty minutes. A convenient schedule is alternating twenty minute periods of application and removal.

Skin and superficial fat is readily cooled by surface cryotherapy, but the effects on deep tissues like muscle and tendon, are somewhat debatable. There is agreement that cooling of underlying muscle requires prolonged exposure exceeding twenty minutes, increasing the risk to the skin. As expected, rewarming of successfully cooled deep tissues takes longer than that of the skin and subcutaneous tissue. Typically, with application of ice, one will experience initial intense cold, then burning sensation, followed by aching and finally, pain relief or anaesthesia (loss of sensation).

As with cold therapy, warm temperature applications have four main effects on body tissues, including pain relief (analgesia), muscle relaxation, blood vessel alterations, and connective tissue relaxation effects. Heat therapy can have both beneficial as well as adverse effects on the tissues, depending upon the magnitude and duration of application. It is not well known how heat administration reduces pain, but perhaps it is by altering pain nerve fibre conduction speeds, or raising nerve pain thresholds. Furthermore, pain secondary to muscle spasm can be alleviated by direct heat application to tender spastic muscle areas. It is wise to wait until after the acute stages of injury and inflammation subside nevertheless, as heat applied early when swelling is prominent can actually increase pain and swelling because of the effects of heat on the blood vessels. Specifically, heat causes a relaxation of blood vessel smooth muscle, thereby opening the vessels and increasing blood flow to the injured region. This phenomenon, combined with direct inflammatory effects, particularly within the skin, mandate a delay in treatment of muscle injury until after swelling resulting from muscle injury has begun to subside. Beneficial effects of increased blood flow to the tissues include facilitation of drainage and a "wash-out" effect, purging the tissues of debris and by-products of tissue injury.

Burns must be avoided when using heat therapy. Therefore, this technique is not to be used where damaged or abnormally sensate skin is present. As mentioned earlier, heat can increase bleeding in the face of very recent soft tissue injury, such as muscle strains, traumatic tendonitis, and ligament sprains. It can also increase joint swelling if injury is acute. Furthermore, heat should probably also be avoided in children and in women during pregnancy.

PULSE

In medicine, a person's pulse is the throbbing of their arteries. It can be palpated in any place that allows for an artery to be compressed against a bone, such as at the neck (carotid artery), at the wrist (radial artery), behind the knee (popliteal artery), on the inside of the elbow (brachial artery), and near the ankle joint (posterior tibial artery). The pulse rate can also be measured by measuring the heart beats directly (the apical pulse).

Pressure waves move the artery walls, which are pliable; these waves are not caused by the forward movement of the blood. When the heart contract, blood is ejected into the aorta and the aorta stretches. At this point, the wave of distention (pulse wave) is pronounced but relatively slow-moving (3-6 m/s). As it travels towards the peripheral blood vessels, it gradually diminishes and becomes faster. In the large arterial branches, its velocity is 7-10 m/s; in the small arteries, it is 15-35 m/s. The pressure pulse is transmitted fifteen or more times more rapidly than the blood flow.

PHYSIOLOGY AND REGULATION

Pulse is also used, though incorrectly, to denote the frequency of the heart beat, commonly measured in beats per minute. In most people, the pulse is an accurate measure of heart rate. Under certain circumstances, including arrhythmias, some of the heart beats are ineffective, and the aorta is not stretched enough to create a palpable pressure wave. The pulse is too irregular and the heart rate can be (much) higher than the pulse rate. In this case, the heart rate should be determined by auscultation of the heart apex, in which case it is not the pulse. The pulse deficit (difference between heart beats and pulsations at the periphery) should be determined by simultaneous palpation at the radial artery and auscultation at the heart apex.

A normal pulse rate for a fit adult, while resting, can range from 60 to 100 beats per minute (BPM), though well-conditioned athletes may have a fit pulse rate lower than 60 BPM. Bradycardia occurs when the pulse rate is below 60 per minute, whereas tachycardia occurs when the rate is above 100 BPM. During sleep, the pulse can drop to as low as 40 BPM; during strenuous exercise, it can rise as high as 150-200 BPM. Generally, pulse rates are higher in infants and young children. The resting heart rate for an infant is commonly close to an adult's pulse rate during strenuous exercise (average 110 BPM for an infant). A collapsing pulse is a sign of hyperdynamic circulation.

CHARACTERISTICS OF THE PULSE

The normal characteristics of the human pulse are volume: the force or strength of the pulse, rhythm: refers to the regularity, or equal spacing of the beats, of the pulse, and the condition of the arterial wall: it should feel elastic and soft.

FACTORS AFFECTING PULSE

- Size: the larger the size, the slower the rate. For instance, a grizzly bear has a heart rate of about 30 beats a minute while a hummingbird's is about 200 beats per minute.
- Gender: a woman's heart rate is generally faster than a man's.

- Age: generally the younger an individual is, the faster the heart rate. An infant's heart rate is about 120 beats per minute; a child's is around 100; an adult's is between 70 and 80; an elderly individual generally hovers in the 60s.
- Exercise: temporarily increases the heart rate.
- Hormones: influence heart rate, especially epinephrine, norepinephrine, and thyroid hormones, all of which can increase the rate.
- Pathology: certain diseases affect heart rate, causing it either to slow or to race. Either one sets the stage for further dysrhythmias.
- Medications and drugs: For instance, digitalis slows the rate, while epinephrine (Adrenalin) increases it. Caffeine can also cause palpitations or extra beats.

ASSESSMENT OF PULSE

1. Evaluate patient for need to monitor pulse because certain diseases or conditions, such as history of heart disease or cardiac dysrhythmias, chest pain, invasive cardiovascular diagnostic tests, infusion of large volume of IV fluids, or haemorrhage, can cause an increased risk for alterations in pulse.
2. Evaluate the pulse for rate, amplitude, contour, and regularity.
3. Evaluate for signs and symptoms of cardiovascular alterations, such as dyspnea, chest pain, orthopnea, syncope, palpitations, edema of extremities, cyanosis, or fatigue, because these signs may indicate deficient cardiac or vascular function.
4. Evaluate patient for components that may affect the character of the pulse, such as age, medications, exercise, change in position, or fever. This enables the nurse to accurately evaluate for the significance of an alteration in pulse.
5. Evaluate for the appropriate site for measuring pulse so that the pulse will be accurate.
6. Evaluate the baseline heart rate and rhythm in the patient's chart to compare it with the current measurement.
7. Evaluate circulatory status by using appropriate site as pulses may be affected by surgery, medical condition, arterial blood draws, or poor circulation.

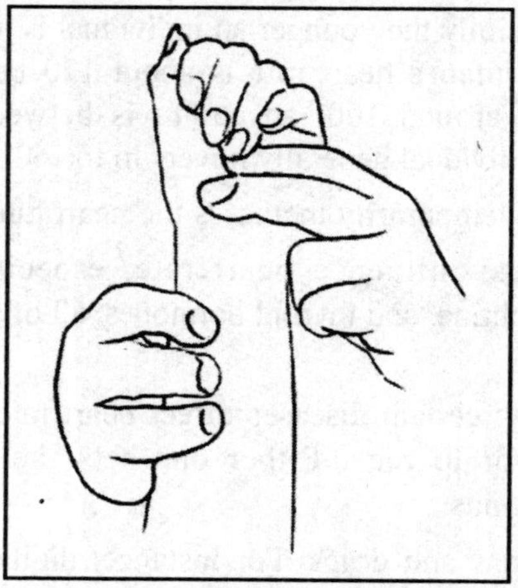

Fig. Taking Pulse

Sites

- Radial - wrist (most common area for taking a pulse)
- Brachial - inner elbow (most common area for taking a blood pressure reading)
- Temporal - temple
- Facial - the cheek just above the jaw near the mouth
- Common carotid - on the neck below the jaw
- Femoral - groin
- Popliteal - behind the knee
- Posterior tibial - just behind the ankle bone
- Dorsalis pedis - top of the foot toward the ankle

Equipments and Techniques

Palpation: Palpation of a pulse involves the index and middle fingers of one hand. Start with gentle pressure to locate the strongest pulsation, and then use firmer palpation for the counting. When counting, also evaluate the rhythm and quality of the pulse. Measure the pulse for 30 and 60 seconds, and then multiply the counts if need be to obtain the one-minute reading.

Auscultation: Auscultation is commonly used to evaluate the apical pulse. The apical pulse is the most accurate pulse, especially when the peripheral pulse is difficult to locate. Auscultation requires the stethoscope. The stethoscope should be equipped with a bell and a diaphragm. The diaphragm side is typically used for low-pitch sound, such as like normal heart sound, bowel sound, or breath sound; the bell side is used for high-pitch sound, such as murmur and abnormal heart sound.

Doppler: An ultrasonic Doppler device is commonly used when the pulse cannot be detected by palpation. The Doppler can detect the peripheral pulses in situations such as cardiopulminary collapse in obese patients, infants with small arms, or patients with edema in which palpation of the pulse is difficult.

The sounds can be amplified and heard through an earpiece or speaker attached to the device, evaluating with low volume initially. Tilt the back of the probe toward the hand at an angle of about 45 degrees. Search the area of the assessed artery and tilt the probe for best Doppler sounds. Adjust the sound volume control to a comfort level for counting.

Special Considerations

Never use the thumb to obtain a pulse because you may sense a beat from your own digital artery that can alter an accurate reading.

When using a Doppler to obtain a foetal heart beat, check the mother's pulse to ensure the beat heard is indeed that of the foetus.

When preparing a patient for surgery related to venous insufficiency of the lower extremities (i.e., femoral-popliteal bypass), it is essential to mark the pedal pulses with an "X." This facilitates locating the pulse during surgery to confirm circulation for the surgeon.

ALTERATIONS IN PULSE

Tremors in geriatric patients can interfere with assessing the radial pulse accurately.

An apical or carotid pulse might be the better option in older patients.

Radial pulses on infants are not reliable because of the small size of the patient and the rapid heart rate normal in infants. A temporal or apical pulse is preferable.

The PMI in an infant is commonly located at the third to fourth intercostal space near the sternum.

A child may be more comfortable sitting on a parent's lap while having his or her pulse assessed.

A curious child may be more cooperative if able to listen to his or her own heart with a stethoscope.

The home care environment can be distracting for the nurse and the patient. The television and loud music can make it difficult to hear an apical pulse and can artificially elevate the patient's pulse rate.

Be sure that the patient is sitting or lying quietly before taking the pulse.

Patients can be taught to evaluate their own pulse, especially when taking cardiac medications.

The relative immobility of most long-term care patients puts them at risk of decreased peripheral circulation. Pedal pulses are an significant part of the nursing examination in long-term-care patients.

RESPIRATION

Passage of respiratory system includes nasal cavity, pharynx, larynx, trachea, bronchioles and alveoli.

Each half of nostril opens into open and atmosphere communicates posteriorly with nasopharynx Nasal epithelium moistens and cleanses the air. Nasal hair are called vibrissal filters macroparticles and don't allow macroparticles to get in while fine particles are trapped along major mucous membrane lining nasal cavity. Second function of nose of medial portion is dealing with olfaction. Third function is of voice phonetics. Paranasal ducts drain into nasal cavity.

PHYSIOLOGY AND REGULATION

Pharynx is about 13 cm long connecting nasal and oral cavity to larynx. Within pharynx lies tonsil. Pharynx has dual role - respiratory as well as digestive.

Nasopharynx has a respiratory function. Uvula a pendulous body hangs from middle lower border of soft palate. Adenoids a collection of lymphoid tissue are situated in the posterior wall of cavity. Oropharanyx is the middle portion. It lies between soft palate and hyoid bone. Adenoids are located along posterior wall and lingual tonsil at the base of the tongue. Larynopharnyx is the lowermost portion of pharynx.

Larynx is a voice box. It checks food or fluid from entering the trachea and lungs during swallowing. Second task of it is to produce sound. It shapes like a triangular box. Thyroid cartilage is known as 'Adam's apple'. Epiglottis is a spoon-shaped cartilage.

The laryngeal muscles are extremely significant in closing the glottis during the act of swallowing and speech too. Mature males generally have thicker and longer vocal cords.

REGULATION OF RESPIRATION

The normal rate of respiration is 14-18 per minute, but the rate and depth of respiration can be adjusted according to the requirement.

The main functions of respiration are to:

i. Supply adequate amount of oxygen

ii. Eliminate CO_2

iii. Regulate H-ion concentration of blood.

iv. Maintain the temperature balance of body.

When metabolic rate increases the need of oxygen increases and eliminates more CO_2. So rate of respiration will increase, while during sleep when BMR is low respiration rate also slows down.

MECHANICS OF BREATHING

Inspiration: It is the process of inhaling air into lungs. During quiet breathing the intrapulmonary pressure decreases about 1 mm Hg below the atmospheric pressure of 760 mm Hg.

Expiration: It is exhalation of air out of lungs. During quiet breathing the intrapulmonary pressure during expiration increases about 1 mm Hg. During forced expiration the volume of thoracic cavity is further reduced by contraction of internal intercostal muscles, which pulls the ribs downwards.

The volume of air that flows is determined by the pressure that moves the air. The relationship between these components can be expressed as:

Pressure = Flow/resistance

CHARACTERISTICS OF THE RESPIRATION

Air always flows from higher pressure to a region of lower pressure. So intrapulmonary pressure should be less than environment. Similarly for air to flow out of the lungs, the intrapulmonary pressure should be more. When the volume of thoracic cavity decreases volume of lung also decreases.

The decrease in lung volume compresses the air within the lungs and intrapulmonary pressure rises above atmospheric pressure. Consequently air flows out of lungs until the pressure within lungs becomes equal to the atmospheric pressure.

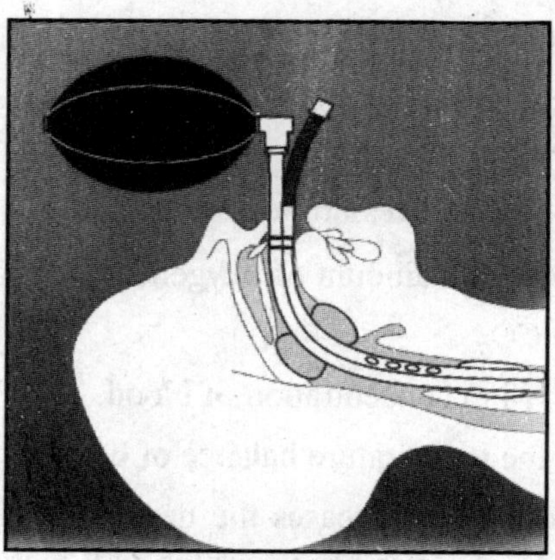

Fig. Artificial respiration

FACTORS AFFECTING RESPIRATION

Acute bronchitis: It is an acute inflammation of the tracheobronchial tree characterized by self-limiting manifestation with cough and fever. It commonly occurs in winter. There will be slight sore throat, irritation, non-productive cough with retrosternal pain. Expetoration may be streaked with blood. Condition runs a course of 7 to 10 days.

Bronchiectasis: It is a chronic disorder with dilatation and destruction of the bronchi. It is characterized by cough with large expectoration of purulent sputum and secondary infection. It gives rise to chronic cough, commonly worse in the morning and often induced by postural changes with large amount of purulent and foul sputum. Breathing appears foul after coughing. •

Pneumococcal pneumonia: It is an acute infection of lungs characterized by chills, fever, cough, chest pain, rust coloured sputum and consolidation. Pneumococcal pneumonia is the most common form. Temperature rises to 103°F to 105°F. Condition gives rise to stabbing pain in chest. Antibiotics give relief.

Pulmonary emphysema: There is overdistension and permanent enlargement of air spaces. It may be caused by destruction of alveolar walls, distortion of airways and bacterial infection. There develops progressive exertional dyspnoea and mucoid expectoration. Chest looks barrel shaped.

Pleural effusion: It is a disorder associated with collection of fluid in the pleural space, characterized by dyspnoea and pleural pain. Clinical features include pleural pain, pyrexia, sweats and expectoration. It pushes mediastinum on opposite side.

Bronchial asthma: It is produced by obstruction of airflow through the bronchioles. It results in dyspnoea, wheezing and other symptoms of asthma. It may require glucocorticoid drugs.

ASSESSMENT OF RESPIRATIONS

Physical Assessment: Respiratory System Assessment (Reason: Investigation of shortness of breath, wheeze and cough)

Inspection: As noted above, rate and rhythm of respirations are within normal limits. Respirations are not laboured. Expiratory phase is not prolonged. During inspiration there is no use of accessory neck muscles, nor does the anterior-posterior diameter of thoracic cage of the posterior chest increase.

Palpation: There is no sign of deformity or tenderness as ribs and sternum are palpated. Expansion of both anterior and posterior chest is symmetric.

Percussion: Location and quality of percussion notes over the lung fields are normal for both anterior and posterior chest. Diaphragmatic excursion of posterior chest is equal bilaterally and measures approximately 5 cm.

Auscultation: Breath sounds from anterior and posterior chest exhibit normal characteristics. There is no presence of adventitious sounds.

BLOOD PRESSURE

Blood pressure refers to the force exerted by circulating blood on the walls of blood vessels, and constitutes one of the principal vital signs. The pressure of the circulating blood decreases as blood moves through arteries, arterioles, capillaries, and veins; the term blood pressure generally refers to arterial pressure, i.e., the pressure in the larger arteries, the blood vessels that take blood away from the heart.

PHYSIOLOGY AND REGULATION

Blood pressure measurement is performed during a physical examination, at initial evaluation, and as part of routine vital signs evaluation. Depending on the patient's condition, the blood pressure is measured by either a direct or indirect technique.

The indirect method requires use of the sphygmomanometer and stethoscope for auscultation and palpation as required. The most common site for indirect blood pressure measurement is the patient's arm over the brachial artery. When the patient's condition prevents auscultation of the brachial artery, the nurse should evaluate the blood pressure in the forearm or leg sites. When pressure measurements in the upper extremities are not accessible, the popliteal artery, located behind the knee, is the site of choice.

The nurse can also evaluate blood pressure in other sites, such as the radial artery in the forearm and the posterior tibial or dorsalis pedis artery in the lower leg. Because it is difficult to auscultate sounds over the radial, tibial, and dorsalis pedis arteries, these sites are commonly palpated to obtain a systolic reading.

The direct method requires an invasive procedure in which an intravenous catheter with an electronic sensor is inserted into an artery and the artery-transmitted pressure on an electronic display unit is read.

FACTORS AFFECTING BLOOD PRESSURE

There are many things which contribute to an individual's risk of developing high blood pressure. These things are collectively called "risk components." Many diseases have significant risk components, and high blood pressure is no exception.

- Age: Being older than age 55 is a significant risk component. Simply stated, the odds of developing high blood pressure increase as we get older.
- Ethnicity: Ethnicity and race is associated with a higher risk of developing high blood pressure.
- Gender: At younger ages, women are less likely to develop high blood pressure than men. This risk equalizes later in life, but statistically, women are still less likely to develop high blood pressure, overall.
- Family History: Having a family history of high blood pressure places you in a higher risk category than someone with no family history of high blood pressure. However, what this actually means is still a topic of research. It is clear that family history plays a significant role in determining risk, but there are probably more significant components, and they are under your control.
- Smoking: Smoking is the number one risk component over which you have control. Smoking is such a powerful risk component for so many different human diseases.

- Exercise: A low exercise lifestyle leads to a weak heart, poor exercise tolerance, and obesity. All of which have been implicated in the development of high blood pressure.
- Diet: While there is evidence that specific items, such as salt, can worsen high blood pressure in certain persons, the main impact that diet plays in high blood pressure risk is that it is a big component in how much you weigh.
- Medications and Drugs: Certain medications can cause or worsen high blood pressure, as can a wide variety of street, or "recreational" drugs, like cocaine, crack, and amphetamines ("speed").
- Kidney Problems: The kidneys are very significant regulators of long term blood pressure, and damage to the kidneys - such as can occur from diabetes - almost invariably leads to high blood pressure.
- Other Medical Problems: Hormone imbalances, certain anatomic abnormalities, tumours, and other medical problems can cause a type of high blood pressure known as secondary hypertension.

ASSESSMENT OF BLOOD PRESSURE

1. Evaluate the condition of the potential blood pressure (BP) site so that a site with an injury or surgery proximal to the site can be avoided.
2. Evaluate the artery for any compromise to it so that compressing the artery briefly will not cause decrease in circulation.
3. Evaluate the distal pulse to check if it is intact and palpable.
4. Evaluate the circumference of the extremity for the right size cuff to be used so an accurate reading can be obtained.
5. Evaluate for components that affect blood pressure, such as age, anxiety, fear, medications, smoking, eating, or exercising within 30 minutes prior to blood pressure evaluation, and postural changes so that an accurate reading can be obtained.
6. Determine patient's baseline blood pressure by reading the medical record so that a comparison can be made with each blood pressure reading.

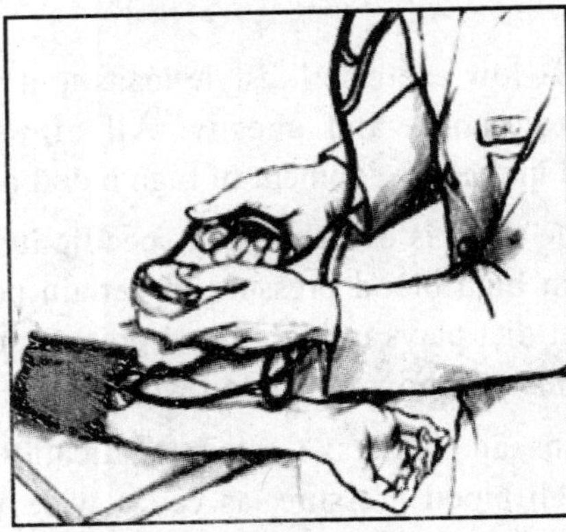

Fig. Measuring Blood Pressure

Sites

The blood pressure must be measured ás close as possible to the aorta, the artery which comes out directly from the heart.

Thus, the reference measurement of the blood pressure is established by a measurement at the level of the artery of the arm (humeral artery), because this artery is the closest to the heart and most easily accessible.

The blood pressure can also be recorded at the level of the arteries of the wrist and even of the fingers. Nevertheless, these sites are by themselves source of error because their distance from the heart is responsible for an artificial rise in the blood pressure.

Moreover, during the measurement, it is very important to place the site of measurement at the level of the heart because gravity is also another source of error.

Indeed, if the subject takes its blood pressure upright, with an outstretched arm along the body, the blood pressure measured at the level of the arm could be raised on an average of 3 millimetres of mercury, whereas if it is measured at the level of the wrist, this increase could be of 15 millimetres of mercury, compared to the blood pressure measured in the aorta!

If the patient is seated, blood pressure variation along the arterial tree is less important, and value of the blood pressure at the brachial site is closed to the value measured at the wrist. For that reason, the device that measure blood pressure at the wrist could perfectly be used in clinical practice.

We thus recommend to choose a self-measurement device of blood pressure, which preferably measures the blood pressure at the level of the arm, or at the wrist, compared to a device measuring the blood pressure at the level the fingers.

Equipments and Techniques

- Stethoscope
- Sphygmomanometer/bladder with mercury column or aneroid dial
- Gloves, if needed
- Alcohol swabs

Mercury Sphygmomanometer: This includes a mercury manometer, an upper arm cuff, a hand inflation bulb with a pressure control valve and requires the use of a stethoscope to listen to the Korotkoff sounds. Relies on the ausculatory technique.

Aneroid Sphygmomanometer: As for a mercury sphygmomanometer, except an aneroid gauge replaces the mercury manometer. The aneroid gauge can be desk mounted or attached to the hand bulb. Again relies on the ausculatory technique.

Semi-automated device: This includes an electronic monitor with a pressure sensor, a digital display, an upper arm cuff and a hand bulb. The pressure is raised manually using the hand bulb. The device automatically deflates the cuff and displays systolic and diastolic values. Pulse rate may also be displayed. Is battery powered and uses the oscillometric technique.

Automated device: This includes an electronic monitor with a pressure sensor, a digital display and an upper arm cuff. An electrically driven pump raises the pressure in the cuff. Devices may have a user-adjustable set inflation pressure or they will automatically inflate to the appropriate level, about 30 mmHg above the predicted systolic reading.

On operation of the start button the device automatically inflates and deflates the cuff and displays the systolic and diastolic values. Pulse rate may so be displayed. Devices may also have a memory facility that stores the last measurement or up to 10 or more previous readings. Is battery powered and uses the ocillometric technique.

Wrist device: This includes an electronic monitor with a pressure sensor, an electrically driven pump and a wrist cuff, or the device itself may be attached to the wrist. Function is similar to the automated device above. Is battery powered and uses the oscillometric technique.

Finger device: This includes an electronic monitor and a finger cuff, or the device itself may be attached to the finger. Is battery powered in general, and uses the oscillometric, pulse-wave or plethysmographic methods.

Automatic Non-Invasive Blood Pressure (NIBP) Monitor: This is a more sophisticated version of the automated device above, with the addition of an automatic-cycling facility to record to the patient's blood pressure at set time intervals. There may also be an option to measure temperature. Alarm limits can commonly be set to alert nursing staff when or more patient functions have exceeded limits. Is mains and battery powered, uses the oscillometric technique.

Ambulatory Blood Pressure Monitor: This includes an upper arm cuff and an electronic monitor with a pressure sensor and an electrically driven pump that attaches to the patient's belt. The unit is programmed to record the patient's blood pressure over a 24-hour period during normal activities and stores the data for future analysis. Is battery powered, and uses ausculatory and oscillometric techniques.

SPECIAL CONSIDERATIONS

Pulsus paradoxus, also called paradoxic pulse, is an abnormal decrease (more than 10 mm Hg) in the systolic pressure and a decrease in pulse wave amplitude during inspiration. An excessive decline may be a sign of tamponade, adhesive pericarditis, severe lung disease, heart failure, or other conditions.

Ask the patient what his or her normal blood pressure is, and use it not only as a gauge for cuff inflation but as an opportunity to teach the patient about fit blood pressure values.

- A child's blood pressure may vary with age. A very low diastolic pressure is not always indicative of underlying cardiac disease.
- An alternative method when taking a blood pressure in a very small infant, when Doppler or automated oscillometric equipment is unavailable, is the flush method, placing a suitable cuff on the arm or leg, raising the limb, and wrapping the extremity distal to the cuff firmly with an elastic bandage until it is drained of blood and blanches. The limb is then lowered to heart level, the cuff is rapidly inflated, and the bandage is removed. As the pressure in the cuff is gradually reduced, flushing of the limb indicates the level at which the flow returns. This level corresponds to mean blood pressure but is inaccurate in infants with anaemia, hypothermia, or edema.

- Blood pressure should be taken in the alternate arm in patients who have recently had a mastectomy with extensive axillary node dissection or other surgical procedure involving the arm or shoulder. In dialysis patients, the alternate arm should be used when the patient has an arteriovenous fistula.

ALTERATIONS IN BLOOD PRESSURE

The systolic blood pressure may be overestimated by the indirect method of measurement because of sclerotic, calcified vessels. If the brachial artery is readily palpable, even when the cuff is inflated and the blood flow is interrupted (positive Olser's sign), then the measurement may not be accurate. Under these circumstances an incorrect diagnosis of hypertension may be made. Direct measurement should be used for confirmation.

Postural hypotension is often observed in the elderly.

Elderly patients may have lost muscle mass, and their upper arms may be quite thin. Be sure to adjust the cuff size to accommodate the patient's arm.

Many elderly patients have a history of hypertension and are taking antihypertensive medications.

Determine the diastolic pressure as Phase IV in children under 13 years of age because the Korotkoff sounds are often heard through the entire period of deflation.

Small children may be uncooperative with the procedure and need the assistance of a parent or adult to hold still.

A cuff that fits adequately may not be available to ensure that the bladder completely encircles the limb. It may be preferable to use the popliteal artery when taking a child's blood pressure.

Blood pressure varies with size as the child reaches adolescence.

REFERENCES

Ackley, B., & Ladwig, G. (1999). Nursing diagnosis handbook: A guide to planning care (4th ed.). St. Louis: Mosby.

Bevis, E. M. (1978). Curriculum building in nursing: A process. St. Louis: Mosby Yearbook.

Brackstone, A. (1993). Rekindling the nursing diagnosis flame. The Canadian Nurse, 89(4), 23–25.

Carlson-Catalano, J. M. (1993). Said another way: What is the language of nursing? Nursing Forum, 28(4), 22–26.

Moss, M. T. (1995). Perioperative nursing in the managed care era: Foundations of nursing empowerment. Nursing Economics, 13(2), 112–114.

Pesut, D., & Herman, J. (1999). Clinical reasoning: The art and science of critical and creative thinking. Albany, NY: Delmar Publishers.

Schaff, A. W. (1990). Meditations for women who do too much. New York: HarperCollins.

Sparks, S., & Taylor, C. (1994). Formulating a nursing diagnosis. Nursing94, 24(3), 32H, 32J.

Thomas, N. M., & Newsome, G. G. (1992). Factors affecting the use of nursing diagnosis. Nursing Outlook, 40(4), 182–186.

Tschikota, S. (1993). The clinical decision-making processes of student nurses. Journal of Nursing Education, 32(9), 389–405.

Whitley, G. (1999). Processes and methodologies for research validation of nursing diagnoses. Nursing Diagnosis, 10(1), 5–13.

8

Assessment of Health

Assessment is the first stage of the nursing process in which the nurse should carry out a complete and holistic nursing evaluation of every patient's needs, regardless of the reason for the encounter. Commonly, an evaluation framework, based on a nursing model is used.

The intention of this stage is to identify the patient's nursing problems. These problems are expressed as either actual or potential. For instance, a patient who has been rendered immobile by a road traffic accident may be assessed as having the "potential for impaired skin integrity related to immobility".

PURPOSE

The assessment is a process during which you use your senses to collect objective data. You will need all of the skills of assessment-cognitive, psychomotor, interpersonal, affective, and ethical/legal-to perform an accurate, thorough physical assessment. You also need to know normal findings before you can begin to distinguish abnormal ones. The best way to perfect your assessment skills is through practice. Effective communication skills are essential to establishing the trust needed to proceed with the examination. Finally, you need to remember your ethical and professional responsibility to your patient in respecting his or her right to privacy and confidentiality.

Assessment provides another perspective. Whereas the health history allows you to see your patient subjectively through hers or his eyes, the examination now allows you to see your patient objectively through your senses. The objective data complete the patient's health picture. Like the health history, the goal of physical assessment is not only to identify actual or potential health problems but also to discover your patient's strengths. Data from the Health assessment can be used to validate the health history. For example, you can use the physical examination to assess clues you obtained from the history.

Combined with the history data, your health assessment findings are essential in formulating nursing diagnoses and developing a plan of care for your patient. Also like the health history, physical assessment may be either complete or focused. A complete physical assessment includes a general survey; vital sign measurements; assessment of height and weight; and physical examination of all structures, organs, and body systems. Perform it when you are examining a patient for the first time and need to establish a baseline. On the other hand, a focused physical assessment zeros in on the acute problem.

You assess only the parts of the body that relate to that problem. It is usually performed when your patient's condition is unstable, as a follow-up to a complete assessment, or when you are pressed for time. The complete physical examination begins with a general survey. A general survey includes your initial observations of the patient's general appearance and behaviour, vital signs, and anthropometric measurements. Vital signs include temperature, pulse, respirations, blood pressure, and pulse oximetry, if available. Anthropometric measurements include height and weight. Next, perform a head-to-toe systematic physical assessment. As you proceed from one area to another, remember that all systems are related, so a problem in one area eventually will affect or be affected by every other system. Therefore, look for the relationships between the systems as you proceed. For example, a skin lesion or a sore that is not healing may be the first sign of an underlying vascular problem or endocrine problem such as diabetes. This assessment can be performed at any level of healthcare prevention-primary, secondary, or tertiary. In a primary setting, a complete physical examination is often

PROCESS OF HEALTH ASSESSMENT

An accurate health assessment requires an organized and systematic approach using the techniques of inspection, palpation, percussion, and auscultation. It also requires a trusting relationship and rapport between the nurse and the patient to decrease the stress the patient may have from being physically exposed and vulnerable. The patient will be much more relaxed and cooperative if you explain what will be done and the reason for doing it. While the findings of a nursing assessment do sometimes contribute to the identification of a medical diagnosis, the unique focus of a nursing assessment is on the patient's responses to actual or potential problems.

The focused health assessment consists of a general survey, vital sign measurements, and assessment of the specific area or system of concern. It also includes a quick head-to-toe scan of the patient, checking for changes in every system as they relate to the problem at hand. This scan may reveal associated problems and help you determine the severity of the problem. For example, if your patient is having breathing problems, do not limit your focused assessment to the respiratory system alone, because detecting confusion or cyanotic skin colour changes may reflect severe hypoxia. The extent of the head-to-toe and focused examinations will depend on your patient's condition and your findings.

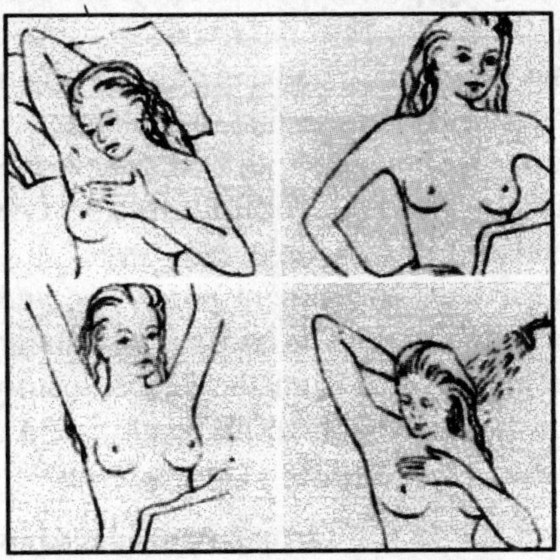

Fig. Self Examination of Breast

A focused physical examination is indicated when your patient's condition is unstable, when time constraints exist, or for episodic follow-up visits. In the last case, you have already performed a complete physical examination, and so now you perform focused physical assessments to monitor or evaluate your patient's health status. Focused physical assessments also can be performed at any level of healthcare prevention. In a primary setting, they may be used to monitor your patient's health status, for example, performing a breast examination and teaching breast self-examination. In a secondary setting, after you have performed the initial physical assessment, focused assessments are often used to monitor and evaluate your patient's health problem. For example, you might take vital signs and then auscultate the lungs of a patient who was admitted with pneumonia. In a long-term-care setting, a focused assessment is often used to monitor and evaluate your patient's progress. For instance, if your patient is recovering from a total hip replacement, you will probably assess his or her musculoskeletal system, including gait, muscle strength, and prescribed range of motion (ROM) of joints.

The physical assessment is the first step in the nursing process. It provides the foundation for the nursing care plan in which your observations play an integral part in the assessment, intervention, and evaluation phases. The chances of overlooking important data are greatly reduced because the physical assessment is performed in an organized, systematic manner, instead of a random manner.

HEALTH HISTORY

The health history provides the subjective database for your evaluation. Often, the health history is your first major interaction with your patient- so make it count. You have only one chance to make a good first impression, and it is often the first impression that your patient will remember. This first encounter provides the foundation and sets the tone for your nurse-patient relationship. The health history is subjective, allowing you to see your patient through his or her "eyes." It comprises of what the patient tells you, what the patient perceives, and what the patient thinks is significant. It provides a holistic, qualitative picture of your patient. Clues that you obtain from the health history will direct your physical evaluation and are essential in developing a successful plan of care for your patient.

The purpose of the health history is to identify not only actual or potential health problems but also your patient's strengths. It should also identify discharge needs. In fact, a successful discharge plan begins on admission with the health history. To create a successful plan of care, you must take a holistic view of your patient and all that affects her or him. Remember: The plan you develop will be successful only if your patient is able to follow through with it after discharge. The purpose of the health history is to:

- Provide the subjective database.
- Identify patient strengths.
- Identify patient health problems, both actual and potential.
- Identify supports.
- Identify teaching needs.
- Identify discharge needs.
- Identify referral needs.

A health history may be either complete or focused. A complete health history includes biographical data, reason for seeking care, current health status, past health status, family history, a detailed review of systems, and a psychosocial profile. A focused health history focuses on an acute problem, so all of your questions will relate to that problem.

COMPLETE HEALTH HISTORY

The complete health history begins with biographical data, including the patient's name, age, gender, birth date, birthplace, marital status, race, religion, address, education, occupation, contact person, and health insurance/social security number. It should also include the source of the health history and his or her reliability, who referred the patient, and whether or not the patient has an advance directive. Once you have obtained this information, you should then identify the reason for seeking healthcare, followed by a description of current health status. The past health history includes childhood illnesses, surgeries, injuries, hospitalizations, adult medical problems, medications, allergies, immunizations, travel, and military service.

The family history will identify familial or genetically linked disorders. The review of systems provides a comprehensive assessment to determine your patient's physiological status. Past or current problems may be identified and warrant further investigation. The psychosocial profile gives you a picture of your patient's health promotion and preventive patterns. It includes a description of health practices and health beliefs, a typical day, nutritional patterns, activity/exercise patterns, recreational patterns, sleep/rest patterns, personal habits, occupational and environmental risk factors, socioeconomic status, developmental level, roles and relationships, self-concept, religious and cultural influences, supports, sexuality patterns, and finally, the emotional health status of your patient. Once you have completed the health history, summarize any pertinent data.

A complete health history provides a comprehensive, holistic picture of your patient. It screens for actual or potential problems and identifies your patient's strengths and health promotion patterns. A complete health history may be obtained in a primary setting as a screening tool, in a secondary setting once your patient's condition stabilizes, or in a tertiary setting to establish a baseline from which to develop your plan of care.

FOCALIZED HEALTH HISTORY

A focalized health history contains necessary biographical data, including the patient's name, age, birth date, birthplace, gender, marital status, dependents, race, religion, address, education, occupation, contact person, and health insurance. It also includes the source of the health history and her or his reliability, who referred the patient, and whether or not the patient has an advance directive. You should then identify the reason for seeking care, followed by a complete symptom analysis. In your past health history, address any areas that relate to the reason for seeking care, including diseases of high incidence, such as heart disease, hypertension, cancer, diabetes, and alcoholism.

In your review of systems, ask questions about every system and how it relates to the presenting health problem. The questions in the psychosocial profile identify the impact of the presenting health problem on your patient's life. A focused health history may be indicated when your patient's condition is unstable or when time constraints are an issue. Focused health histories may also be used for episodic follow-up visits for your patient. In this case, you have already obtained a detailed health history at an earlier point and have established the subjective database. During the follow-up visits, you need to obtain further subjective data to monitor and evaluate your patient's progress. Once you have completed the focused health history, remember to document any pertinent findings.

CONSTITUENTS OF THE HEALTH HISTORY

A complete health history addresses health and illness patterns, health promotion and protective patterns, and roles and relationships. The parts of the health history that focus on health and illness patterns include the biographical data, reason for seeking healthcare, current health status, past health history, family history, and review of systems. You identify not only current health problems but also past health problems and any familial factors that place your patient at risk for health problems. Your patient's health promotion activities, protective patterns, and role and relationship patterns are assessed through the psychosocial component of the health history. Here, you assess for risk factors that pose a threat to your patient's health in every aspect of her or his life. Also, you need to consider your patient's cultural and developmental status as it affects her or his health status.

Biographic Data

The biographical data provide you with direct information related to a current health problem, alert you to risk factors for health problems, and point out the need for referrals. Your patient's ability to provide biographical data accurately reflects his or her mental status. Biographical data include the patient's name, address, phone number, contact person, age/birth date, place of birth, gender, race, religion, marital status, educational level, occupation, and health insurance. They also include the person who provided the history and her or his reliability as well as the person who referred the patient. Information on advance directives may also be obtained for hospital admissions. Also note any special considerations, such as the use of an interpreter.

Grounds for Seeking Healthcare

Ask your patient why he or she is seeking healthcare; then document his or her direct quote. The patient's reason for seeking care is usually related to the level of preventive healthcare -primary, secondary, or tertiary. If the setting is a primary level of healthcare, there is usually no acute problem. The reason generally relates to health maintenance or promotion. For example, the patient states, "I am here for my annual physical examination." If there is an acute problem, ask the patient to state what the problem is and how long it has been going on. For example, "I have had chest pain for the last hour." If your patient identifies more than one problem, she or he may be confusing associated symptoms with the primary problem.

Help her or him clarify and prioritize the problems by asking questions such as, "Which problems are giving you the most difficulty?" Usually, patients identify problems that affect their ability to do what they usually do. In an acute-care setting, the reason for seeking care is called the chief complaint. The chief complaint gives you the patient's perspective on the problem, a view of the problem through his or her eyes. At the tertiary level, the problem may be well defined, a chronic problem, or an acute problem that is resolving. In this case, the problem does not have the acuity or life-threatening urgency of an acute problem.

Present Health Condition

Once you have identified the patient's reason for seeking healthcare, assess her or his current health status. At a primary level of healthcare (no acute problem), the current health status should include the following:

- Any health concerns. For example: Patient is Usha Gupta, age 42, married, mother of three, full-time teacher. Usual state of health good. Has yearly physical with pelvic examination and dental examination. Last eye examination 1 year ago. Expresses concern regarding family history of hypertension and ovarian cancer.
- Any major health problems.
- Usual patterns of healthcare.
- Usual state of health.

Patients in secondary or tertiary healthcare settings have an existing problem. So you will need to perform a symptom analysis to assess your patient's presenting symptoms thoroughly. Although many questions come to mind, your patient's condition and time constraints may preclude you from going into too much detail. If so, you'll need to zero in on several key areas to evaluate your patient's symptoms. As you perform the symptom analysis, try to determine how disabling this problem is for your patient. Also ask if he or she has any medical problems related to the current problems and if he or she is taking any medications for this current problem.

PHYSICAL EXAMINATION

A physical examination is an assessment of the body and its functions using inspection, palpation (feeling with the hands), percussion (tapping with the fingers), and auscultation (listening). A complete health evaluation also includes gathering information about a person's medical history and lifestyle, doing laboratory tests, and screening for disease.

METHODS

The four techniques of physical evaluation are inspection, palpation, percussion, and auscultation. They are performed in this order, with the exception of the abdominal evaluation. In this case, auscultation precedes palpation and percussion so as not to alter the bowel sounds.

Inspection: Always begin with inspection. Inspection is the most frequently used evaluation technique, but its value is often overlooked. With inspection, you use not only your sense of sight but also your senses of hearing and smell to inspect your patient critically. Do not rush the process; take your time and really look at your patient. Perform inspection at every encounter with your patient. Be sure you have adequate lighting, and sufficiently expose the area being assessed. Be systematic in your approach, working from head to toe and noting key landmarks and normal findings. Use your patient as a comparative when possible. Ask yourself, "Does it look the same on the left side as the right?" Look for surface characteristics such as colour, size, and shape. Ask yourself, "Are there colour changes? Is the patient symmetrical?" Look for gross abnormalities or signs of distress. Do you notice any unusual odours or hear any unusual sounds that warrant further investigation? Always view your findings in light of the patient's growth and developmental stage and cultural background, which may influence your interpretation. For instance, an older patient with acute appendicitis may not present with acute abdominal pain as is seen in a younger patient, or a patient with the same problem may not complain of severe pain since pain is something to be endured in his or her culture.

Inspection may be direct or indirect. Direct inspection involves directly looking at your patient. Indirect inspection involves using equipment to develop visualization. For instance, the oto/ophthalmoscope allows better visualization of the ears and eyes; and specula, such as the nasal speculum and vaginal speculum, open and illuminate, allowing for better visualization.

PREPARATION FOR EXAMINATION

The client and the environment require special consideration. Because the client will experience some anxieties regarding the examination, it is important for the nurse to keep the client informed while performing the examination. The nurse needs to be organized and demonstrate respect for the client's apprehension about physical exposure during the examination. Although some uneasiness may be experienced when learning how to perform a physical examination, it is important that the nurse appear calm, organized, and competent at the bedside. Review the agency's physical examination/assessment form before meeting with the client. This process ensures that the nurse can fully explain the actions that will be performed and prevents omission of any area required to be assessed. The nurse usually takes the assessment form to the bedside to record the data to ensure accuracy of documentation.

Environment

The nurse should review the health and psychosocial assessment data before visiting the client so that the environment will accommodate any special needs of the client. Adjust the environment to allow for placement of the equipment on a surface that is clean and free from movement at the bedside. Check to make sure that nothing is on the floor that would place the client at risk for falling. The room needs to be quiet, warm, without drafts, and adequately lit. Depending on the setting, make the necessary adjustments to ensure privacy. Inform other personnel about the time of the examination to avoid interruptions, which are frustrating to both the client and the nurse.

Equipment

Wash hands and gather the necessary equipment. The nurse should review the protocol relative to a physical examination and secure the forms required for documenting the assessment findings. Secure enough clean gloves to change as needed throughout the examination to avoid cross-contamination.

Positioning and Draping

The nurse should position the client to ensure accessibility to the body part being assessed. The primary purpose of draping the client is to prevent unnecessary exposure during the examination. Feelings of embarrassment elicit tension and restlessness and will decrease the client's ability to cooperate. The drapes also prevent the client from being chilled. The drape may be cloth or paper; for example, a bath blanket, sheet, or towel. The client's gown can be rearranged to expose and cover different body parts. When the client is in a sitting, supine, dorsal recumbent, Sims', or prone position, use a gown or towel to cover the upper chest and a bath blanket or sheet to cover the rest of the body. Although you will not be expected to place the client in the lithotomy position to conduct an internal vaginal examination, you may be expected to assist another practitioner with this examination. Draping a client in the lithotomy position requires a sheet and boots. The nurse should apply the boots, if available, to cover each of the client's feet and legs. Fold and place the sheet in a diamond-shaped arrangement over the body: top diamond under chin with opposite corner pointing toward the toes and lateral corners pointing toward the sides of the table. Ask the client to flex her knees, and with the lateral corners of the sheet, wrap it in a spiral fashion around the legs and feet. The bottom corner covers the perineum and is folded back over the abdomen to expose the perineum when the examination begins.

GENERAL ASSESSMENT

Always begin the physical evaluation with the general survey. This "first impression" of your patient begins as soon as you meet him or her. Use your senses and your observational skills to look, listen, and take note of any unusual odours. First, look for the obvious: apparent age, gender, and race. Then look closer for clues that might signal a problem. Also consider your patient's developmental stage and cultural background; these may influence your findings and interpretation. Make a mental note of any clues detected on the general survey that you may need to follow up during the physical examination. When looking for clues, watch for signs of distress and check facial characteristics, body size and type, posture, movements, speech, grooming, dress, and hygiene.

ASSESSMENT OF EACH BODY SYSTEM

With the individual being examined in a sitting position, the following systems are reviewed:

- Skin: The exposed areas of the skin are observed; the size and shape of any lesions are noted.
- Head: The hair, scalp, skull, and face are examined.
- Eyes. The external structures are observed. The internal structures can be observed using an ophthalmoscope (a lighted instrument) in a darkened room.
- Ears: The external structures are inspected. A lighted instrument called an otoscope may be used to inspect internal structures.
- Nose and sinuses. The external nose is examined. The nasal mucosa and internal structures can be observed with the use of a penlight and a nasal speculum.
- Mouth and pharynx: The lips, gums, teeth, roof of the mouth, tongue, and pharynx are inspected.
- Neck: The lymph nodes on both sides of the neck and the thyroid gland are palpated.
- Back: The spine and muscles of the back are palpated and checked for tenderness. The upper back, where the lungs are located, is palpated on the right and left sides and a stethoscope is used to listen for breath sounds.
- Breasts and armpits: A woman's breasts are inspected with the arms relaxed and then raised. In both men and women, the lymph nodes in the armpits are felt with the examiner's hands. While the individual is still sitting, movement of the joints in the hands, arms, shoulders, neck, and jaw can be checked.

While the individual is lying down on the examining table, the examination includes:

- Breasts: The breasts are palpated and inspected for masses.
- Front of chest and lungs: The area is inspected with the fingers, using palpation and percussion. A stethoscope is used to listen to internal breath sounds.

The head should be slightly raised to examine:

- Heart: A stethoscope is used to listen to the heart's rate and rhythm. The blood vessels in the neck are observed and palpated.
- The individual being examined should lie flat for an examination of the:

- Abdomen: Light and deep palpation is used on the abdomen to feel the outlines of internal organs, including the liver, spleen, kidneys, and aorta, a large blood vessel.
- Rectum and anus: With the individual lying on the left side, the outside areas are observed. An internal digital examination (using a gloved finger), is commonly done for persons over 40 years old. In men, the prostate gland is also palpated.

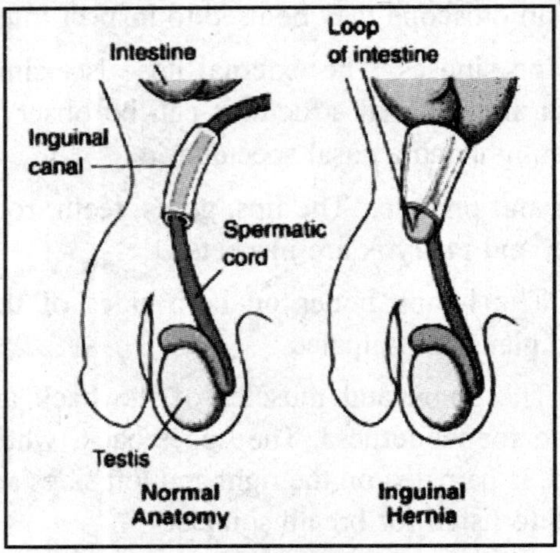

Fig. Inguinal Hernia

- Reproductive organs: The external sex organs are inspected and the area is examined for hernias. In men, the scrotum and testicles are palpated. In women, a pelvic examination is completed using a speculum and a sample for a Papanicolaou test (Pap test) may be taken.
- Legs: While lying flat, the legs are inspected for swelling, and pulses in the knee, thigh, and foot area are found. The groin area is palpated for the presence of lymph nodes. The joints and muscles are observed.
- Musculoskeletal system: With the individual standing, the straightness of the spine and the alignment of the legs and feet are noted.
- Blood vessels: The presence of any abnormally enlarged veins (varicose), commonly in the legs, is noted.

In addition to assessing a person's alertness and mental ability during the initial conversation, inspection of the nervous system may include:

- Neurological screen: The person's ability to take a few steps, hop, and do deep knee bends is observed. The strength of the handgrip is felt. While sitting in an upright position, the reflexes in the knees and feet can be tested with a small hammer. The sense of touch in the hands and feet can be evaluated by testing reaction to pain and vibration.
- The 12 nerves in the head (cranial) that are connected directly to the brain. They control the senses of smell and taste, strength of muscles in the head, reflexes in the eye, facial movements, gag reflex, vision, hearing, and muscles in the jaw. General muscle tone and coordination, and the reaction of the abdominal area to stimulants like pain, temperature, and touch may also be evaluated.

VARIATIONS IN EXAMINATION TECHNIQUES FOR DIFFERENT AGES

For patients of different ages, following points should be kept in mind:

- Chief complaint: reason for seeking medical attention; when possible it should be stated in the patient's own words.
- Present illness: chronologic narrative of the patient's medical problems. The description of the symptoms should include the following: location, radiation, quality (deep, sharp, stinging), quantity or severity, timing (onset, duration, frequency), aggravating or relieving factors, associated manifestations, prior investigations, prior treatment.
- Past medical history: general state of health, significant childhood and adult illnesses, prior hospitalizations (medical, surgical).
- Current medications: dose frequency and duration of present drug regimen; include all non-prescription drugs.
- Family history: age and health status or age and cause of death of each immediate family member. Inquire about a family history of diabetes, heart disease, hypertension cancer, arthritis, mental disorders, or any hereditary conditions.

REVIEW OF SYSTEMS

- General: overall state of health, usual weight, recent weight change, fever, night sweats, sleeping habits, appetite

- Skin: rashes, pruritus, colour change, pigmentation
- Head: headaches, trauma
- Eyes: vision, visual disturbances, last eye examination
- Ears: hearing, tinnitus, vertigo, infections, discharge
- Nose and sinuses: epistaxis, nasal stuffiness, sinusitis, sense of smell
- Mouth and throat: condition of teeth, last dental examination, complaints of sore throat or mouth lesions
- Neck: lumps, "swollen glands," pain in the neck region
- Breast: pain, history of lumps, bleeding, nipple discharge; if female, inquire if patient performs self-examination
- Respiratory: cough, wheezing, sputum (quantity, colour), shortness of breath, pain associated with breathing
- Cardiac: chest pain, palpitations, orthopnea, edema, heart murmurs, history of high blood pressure
- Gastrointestinal: nausea, vomiting, change in bowel habits, gastrointestinal bleeding, constipation, diarrhoea, abdominal pain, increased girth
- Genitourinary: dysuria, frequency, urgency, nocturia, discharges, sexually transmitted diseases (STDs), libido, sexual problems, bleeding
- Gynaecologic/reproductive: age at menarche, last menstrual period, frequency and duration of menses, number and complications of pregnancies, age at menopause, contraception
- Musculoskeletal: weakness, arthritis, gout, joint pains, swelling or stiffness, muscle cramps
- Peripheral vascular: varicose veins, thrombophlebitis, claudication, Raynaud's phenomenon
- Neuropsychiatry: seizures, syncope, weakness, paralysis, extreme mood changes, insomnia, anxiety, psychiatric care, suicidal ideation
- Endocrine: heat or cold intolerance, polydypsia, polyuria, polyphagia
- Haematology: easy bruising, transfusion reactions, excessive bleeding, history of anaemia

REFERENCES

Alfaro-LeFevre, R. (1997). Applying nursing process: A stepby- step guide (3rd ed.). Philadelphia: Lippincott.

Alfaro-LeFevre, R. (1998). Critical thinking in nursing: A practical approach (2nd ed.). Philadelphia: Saunders.

Arnold, E., & Boggs, K. (1999). Interpersonal relationships: Professional communication skills for nurses (3rd ed.). Philadelphia: Saunders.

Bloom, B. (Ed.). (1956). Taxonomy of educational objectives, handbook I: Cognitive domain. New York: David McKay.

Carpenito, L. J. (1999a). Handbook of nursing diagnosis (8th ed.). Philadelphia: Lippincott.

Carpenito, L. J. (1999b). Nursing care plans and documentation: Nursing diagnosis and collaborative problems (3rd ed.). Philadelphia: Lippincott.

Grant, J. (1999). Objectives, goals, and outcomes: What's the difference? Home Healthcare Nurse, 17(5), 284–286.

Hansten, R., & Washburn, M. (1999). Seven steps to shift from tasks to outcomes. Nursing Management, (30)7, 35–37.

Johnson, M., Maas, M., & Moorhead, S. (Eds.). (1999). Nursing outcomes classification (NOC). St. Louis: Mosby.

Maas, M. L, & Johnson, M. (Eds.). (1997). Nursing outcomes classification (NOC): Iowa outcomes project. St. Louis: Mosby.

Oermann, M. H., & Huber, D. (1999). Patient outcomes: A measure of nursing's value. American Journal of Nursing, 99(9), 40–47.

Sparks, S. M., & Taylor, C. M. (1993). Nursing diagnosis reference manual (2nd ed.). Springhouse, PA: Springhouse.

9

Needs of Patient

Health is one of our most precious possessions. The preservation of health is met through the satisfaction of our basic human needs. Understanding the basic needs of people, therefore, is essential for the practical nurse in planning for and meeting the needs of the patient.

The individual's state of health is one of continual change. He moves back and forth from health to illness and back to health again. His condition is rarely constant. He may wake up feeling great, develop a headache mid-morning, and feel fine again by noon. The health-illness continuum illustrates this process of change, in which the individual experiences various states of health and illness (ranging from extremely good health to death) that fluctuate throughout his life.

Health, just as life itself, is a process of continual change. And we must continually adapt to these changes in our lives in order to maintain good health and well-being. It is our adaptation or response to that change, rather than the change itself, that affects our health. For example, two students just found out about a big test tomorrow, for which they are completely unprepared. One student responds to this stressful situation (stressor) by going home, getting his books out, and starting to study. The other student breaks out into a sweat, and spends most of the evening fretting over this outrage and imagining what will happen to him if he doesn't pass the test. No doubt, this student is doing more damage to his health than is his friend. And, considering the time and energy he is expending on worrying (and not studying), he may experience even more stress when they receive their grades.

BASIC HUMAN NEEDS

Physical Needs: These are closely related to body functions and are sometimes referred to as primary or physiological drives. Physical needs include:

- Food.
- Water.
- Oxygen.
- Elimination.
- Clothing and shelter for body warmth and protection.
- Activity, or sensory and motor stimulation, including sex, physical exercise, and rest.

Emotional Needs: Emotional needs are closely interwoven with physical needs and are met in interaction with significant others. They include:

- Love, including approval and esteem.
- Importance, including recognition and respect. This applies to the patient's perception of the nurse's feelings toward him. For example, if your patient feels that you do not approve of or respect him, he may become very demanding, or he may withdraw and not cooperate with your efforts to make him healthy again.
- Adequacy, including self-sufficiency and the need to be needed and wanted.
- Productivity, including work and creative pursuits.

Social Needs: Social needs grow out of the culture and society of which one is a member. They include:

- Identification or belonging.
- Education or learning.
- Recreation or play.
- Religion or worship.

MASLOW'S HIERARCHY OF NEEDS

Psychologist Abraham Maslow defined basic human needs as a hierarchy, a progression from simple physical needs to more complex emotional needs. Types of Needs are:

- Physiological: food, shelter, water, sleep, oxygen.
- Safety: security, stability, order, physical safety.
- Love and belonging: affection, identification, companionship.
- Esteem and recognition: self-esteem, self-respect, prestige, success, esteem of others.

- Self-actualization: self-fulfillment, achieving one's own capabilities.
- Aesthetic: beauty, harmony, spiritual.

Remember that human needs are not constant; they are fluid and changing with first one, then another, taking priority. What may start as a basic need for food can take on social and personal significance. Your care plan as well as your patience are aimed toward the satisfaction of the patient's needs. He has common needs because he is a person; he has individual needs because he is unique; he has special needs because he is sick. The Practical Nurse supplies the help that is required to meet the patient's needs during the stressful periods of hospitalization and recuperation.

SAFE ENVIRONMENT

Safe care is a basic need of all clients regardless of the setting. Nurses are responsible for providing the client with a safe environment through the delivery of professional, quality nursing care that incorporates safety precautions, infection control practices, and hygiene assistance. This chapter describes the nurse's role in each of these areas. Safety has a positive association with health promotion and illness prevention. A safe environment reduces the risk of accidents, subsequent alterations in health and lifestyle, and the cost of health care services. There are many factors in the environment that can threaten safety.

Nurses provide and maintain a safe and clean environment in health care facilities. They provide fundamental patient care, which includes answering call signals and supplying and emptying bed pans. They provide patients with assistance in activities of daily living, such as bathing, dressing and grooming. Sometimes they serve meal trays and feed patients. To help patients recover, they lift, turn or massage patients, and they may also supervise patients' exercise routines. As directed by nursing and hospital staff, they take fundamental measurements, such as patients' blood pressure, temperature and pulse. They collect specimens, such as urine, faeces or sputum, administer suppositories, colonic irrigations and enemas, and perform other procedures. They transport patients in wheelchairs or stretchers for treatment or surgery, carry messages, reports, requisitions and specimens from one department to another, and maintain an inventory of supplies. In acute care as well as in long term care settings, orderlies perform nursing procedures, such as catheterization and sterile dressings.

FACTORS AFFECTING SAFETY

Client safety is influenced by several factors such as age, lifestyle, sensory and perceptual alterations, mobility, and emotional state.

Age

Risk for injury varies with chronological age and developmental stage. Health education about preventive measures can facilitate injury prevention for various age groups. As infants mature, their potential for injury increases. Infants, toddlers, and preschoolers are explorers of their environment. Most accidents involving these age groups are preventable with careful adult supervision to prevent falls from bed, burns, electrical hazards, choking on small objects, and drowning.

As school-age children explore their environment outside the home, their risk for injury increases. Prevention measures during this stage focus on not accepting candy, food, gifts, or rides from strangers; bicycle, skating, and swimming safety; and substance abuse. Adolescents and young adults usually enjoy good physical health; however, their lifestyles put them at risk for injury. Since this age group spends much time away from home, collaborative educational efforts among parents, schools, and community health care providers need to focus on environmental safety.

High-risk factors for this age group include fatigue, anxiety, sleep pattern disturbances, caregiver role strain, and altered health maintenance. The older adult is prone to falls, especially in the bathroom, bedroom, and kitchen, because of a loss of agility and visual acuity, predisposition to dizziness and syncope, and side effects of medications. Prevention measures for this age group emphasize slow position changes, good lighting, hand rails, and skidproof strips in the bathtub or shower and under rugs and carpets. Each year, approximately one-third of people over the age of 65 who live at home fall; 15% of falls cause serious injuries, half of which are fractures.

Lifestyle

Lifestyle practices can increase a person's risk for injury and potential for disease. Individuals who operate machinery; experience stress, anxiety, and fatigue; use alcohol and drugs (prescription and non-prescription); and live in high-crime neighbourhoods are at risk for injury. Risk-taking behaviours such as daredevil activities, driving vehicles at high speeds, and smoking are factors associated with accidents.

Sensory and Perceptual Alterations

Sensory functions are essential for accurate perception of environmental safety. If one of the senses is altered, then the other senses compensate to facilitate perception of the environment. For instance, a blind person usually will develop a keen sense of touch and hearing. Clients who have visual, hearing, taste, smell, communication, or touch perception impairments are at increased risk for injury. These clients are often not able to perceive a potential danger.

Mobility

Clients who have impaired mobility are at increased risk for injury, especially falls. Mobility impairments may be a result of poor balance or coordination, muscle weakness, or paralysis. Immobility may also precipitate physiological and emotional complications such as decubitus and depression, respectively.

Emotional State

Emotional states such as depression and anger affect a client's perception of environmental hazards and degree of risk-taking behaviour. These emotional states alter a client's thinking patterns and reaction time. Usual safety precautions may be forgotten during periods of emotional stress. Self-confidence decreases when an elderly person falls; they tend to limit their activities because they fear falling again.

REDUCTION OF PHYSICAL HAZARDS

Bathroom Hazards

Bathrooms pose a threat to the client in the home because of the presence of water and storage of medication. Common bathroom accidents are falls, scalds or burns, and poisonings. Bathroom accidents can be reduced by the use of grab bars near the tub, shower, and toilet; nonslip mats in the tub and shower; and a secured bathroom rug near the tub or shower. Other safety measures include checking the temperature of the water before entering tub or shower; checking the thermostat setting on the water heater; and storing medications in a locked cabinet, out of reach of children or disoriented or confused adults.

Fire

Fire is a potential danger to all people in an institutional or home environment. Immobilized or incapacitated clients are at increased risk during a fire. Common causes of fire are smoking in bed, discarding cigarette butts in trash cans, and faulty electrical equipment. Fire occurs with the interaction of three elements: sufficient heat to ignite the fire, combustible material, and oxygen to support the fire. Nursing goals are fire prevention and protection of clients during a fire. Nursing interventions aimed at preventing or reducing the risk of fire includes:

- Checking electrical cords and outlets for exposed or damaged wires
- Clearly marking fire exits
- Educating clients about fire hazards In the event of a fire, follow institutional policy and procedures for fire containment and evacuation.
- Keeping open spaces and hallways clear of clutter
- Knowing locations of fire extinguishers and their operation
- Posting emergency phone numbers by all telephones
- Practicing fire evacuation procedures
- Reporting identified electrical hazards

Nursing interventions during a fire are directed at protecting the client from injury and containing the fire. Nurses should be familiar with the location of fire alarm pull boxes. If a fire occurs, the nurse should utilize the nearest fire box for notification and move clients to safety. Nurses should be familiar with the use of fire extinguishers and their locations. The fire extinguisher should be directed toward the base of the fire. The four types of fire extinguishers used are water, carbon dioxide, regular dry chemical, and multipurpose dry chemical. Each type of fire extinguisher is used for a specific class of fire.

Electrical Equipments

Clients have contact with a variety of electrical equipment in the hospital environment, such as bed controls and intravenous and patient-controlled analgesia (PCA) pumps. All electrical equipment should have a three pronged electrical plug that is grounded. A grounded plug transmits any stray electrical current from equipment to the ground. To protect the client from electrical injury, the nurse should read the warning labels on all equipment, use only grounded electrical equipment, check for frayed electrical cords, avoid overloading circuits, and report any shocks received from equipment to the biomedical department. If a client receives an electrical shock, the nurse should turn off or remove the electric source before touching the client. Then, the client's pulse should be checked. If the client has no pulse, CPR should be initiated. If the client has a pulse, the nurse should assess vital signs, mental status, and skin integrity for burns. A physician should be notified of the event. The nurse should note points of entry and exit of electrical current to assess for potential complications.

Exposure to Radiation

Clients are exposed to radiation during diagnostic testing and therapeutic interventions. Injury can occur from radiation if there is overexposure or exposure to untargeted tissues. Exposure to untargeted tissues can occur with radiation implants that become dislodged. General principles of radiation exposure and protection are based on time, distance, and shielding. Protection from radiation therapy includes:

- Labelling all potentially radioactive material
- Maximizing distance from radiation source (implants or client)
- Minimizing time in contact with radiation source (implants or client)
- Monitoring radiation exposure with a film badge
- Never touching dislodged implants or body fluids of client.
- Using appropriate radiation shields

The client's risk for injury can be reduced by educating the client about radiation treatment and necessary precautions, placing the client in a private room, and providing a lead apron when necessary to protect non targeted body tissues. The nurse's risk for injury can be reduced by observing all radioactive labels, wearing gloves when handling radioactive body discharges, washing hands, wearing lead aprons, disposing of radioactive substances in special containers, reducing time of client contact, and wearing badges that measure the amount of radiation exposure.

Poisoning

A poison is any substance that causes an alteration in the client's health, such as injury or death, when inhaled, injected, ingested, or absorbed by the body. Antidotes and treatments are available for some but not all types of poisonings. Direct and indirect causes of poisonings are:

- Improper storage of toxic substances
- Inadequate supervision of children
- Ingestion of household plants

- Insect or snake bites
- Accidental ingestion of a toxic substance or medication overdose

The poison control centre should be notified when poisoning is suspected. The person reporting the poisoning should be prepared to state the amount and type of poison ingested, inhaled, or injected, client's age, and symptoms. Clients who have ingested poison should be turned on their side to prevent aspiration while awaiting further treatment. Client education about safety measures can prevent some accidental poisonings.

Noise Pollution

Noise pollution, a situation that results when the noise level becomes uncomfortable for the client or staff, frequently occurs in the health care setting as a result of visitor traffic, medical equipment, and personnel. It can result in an unorganized environment, hearing loss, and sensory overload. Sensory overload is an increased perception of the intensity of auditory and visual stimuli. Sensory overload can alter a client's recovery by increasing anxiety, paranoia, hallucinations, and depression. Safety measures include maintaining a quiet environment, traffic control, and providing earplugs.

SAFETY DEVICES

Restraints

Restraints are protective devices used to limit the physical activity of a client or to immobilize a client or extremity. Restraints are used to protect the client, allow for treatment in a safe environment, and reduce the risk of injury to others. The use of restraints has become very controversial because of client injuries from restraints. Nurses must document, according to the institutional protocol, the application and care of the client in restraints. Restraints used to either limit physical activity or immobilize a client can be physical or chemical.

Physical restraints reduce the client's movement through the application of a device. Most states require a physician's order for the application of physical restraints.

Chemical restraints are medications used to control the client's behaviour. Commonly used chemical restraints are anxiolytics and sedatives.

Common types of physical restraints are:

- Belt: Straps or belts applied across the client to secure him or her to the stretcher, bed, or wheelchair.

- Elbow: A combination of fabric and plastic or wooden tongue blades that immobilize the elbow to prevent flexion.
- Jacket (body restraint): A sleeveless vest with straps that cross in front or back of the client and are tied to the bed frame or chair legs.
- Limb or extremity: Cloth devices that immobilize one or all limbs by securely tying the restraint to the bed frame or chair.
- Mitten or hand: Enclosed cloth material applied over the client's hand to prevent injury from scratching.
- Mummy: A blanket or sheet that is folded around the child to limit movement. Mummy restraints are used to perform procedures on children. The nursing plan of care should include safety measures to reduce the potential for injury from restraints. Additional safety measures to observe when using restraint devices are:

Restraints can be changed and released easily, using only a clove hitch knot.

Restraints should not interfere with any treatments (e.g., intravenous therapy) or aggravate the client's health problem.

There should be enough slack on the straps so that the client can move both arms and legs and for range-of-motion exercises.

At least once every 2 hours, the nurse must perform circulation and neurological exams, assessing the colour, sensation, temperature, motion, and capillary refill in the area distal to the restraint.

There should be a provision for psychological support of client and significant others. The restraint strap is secured to the bed frame, not to the side rail so as to avoid accidental injury to the extremity in the event that the side rail is released while the restraint strap is attached to it.

Removing Obstacles

Obstacles in heavily travelled areas of health care facilities or homes are a risk to the client's safety. Older adults or persons who are unfamiliar with the environment are at greatest risk of injury from obstacles. The risk that obstacles pose can be reduced by keeping hallways clear, removing excess furniture from heavily travelled areas, removing all electrical cords or taping cords securely to the floor, removing throw rugs, applying nonslip pads to rugs, cleaning up spills immediately, and removing objects that could fall from the tops of appliances.

ROLE OF NURSE IN PROVIDING SAFE AND CLEAN ENVIRONMENT

There is a direct connection between nursing actions and the health of the environment in health care agencies. However, in daily practice nurses, whether administering a medication, changing a dressing, or starting an IV, do not commonly consider the environmental impact of such activities. For instance, discarding wrappers that represent by-products of their work is an almost subliminal activity in their professional role since their focus as a nurse is more frequently on other priorities. To recognize the unconscious nature of many of nursing activities that do impact the environment, such as waste disposal, nurses need to take a moment and reflect on the last time they worked. It helps to do an evaluation of the many items handled in a given shift that could have a negative effect on the environment.

To do an adequate evaluation of the impact of nursing care on the environment, one must consider everything in the environment including the lighting, air conditioning or heating, electrical equipment and pumps, elevators, computers, electronic medication dispensing machines, monitors, and more. This exercise reveals the environmental infrastructure of health care and displays the 'ecological footprint' of health care, which is a metaphor used to depict the resources a person, institution, or community would hypothetically need to support itself and to absorb its wastes, given the known technology. Such reflection utilizes the fundamental skills of inquiry nurses use every day with patients and allows them to establish a holistic view of the conditions in their place of work that may need remediation.

However, nurses seldom do such evaluations because environmental systems are generally silent partners in the work they do. It is only when systems break down that an environmental problem becomes obvious. It is only when waste containers overflow that one thinks about them. When bags of waste disappear without clinicians being aware of these bags, they do not think about where that waste goes. Until recently the disposal and treatment of infectious and hazardous chemical wastes from health care was a foremost contributor of dioxin and mercury pollution. Even today health care wastes remain a public health and an environmental problem.

Nurses make numerous waste disposal and material use decisions daily, decisions that can affect the health of our environment. They need to become and remain informed regarding the policies related to hospital environmental health and general state of the environmental health of their own institutions. Furthermore, they need to take a foremost role in promoting the environmental health of their health care agencies. Key steps nurses can take to fulfill this role include:

- Meeting with the organization's environmental services or environmental health and safety division to ensure that there is an effective process of sharing the most up-to-date environmental safety information and waste management policies with nursing
- Mastering and using environmental rules, leveraging the need to be in perpetual, inspection readiness mode as a way of expediting compliance with safety regulations.
- Recommending the hospital join in with the "greening" of health care movement, and utilizing the partnership and recognition award opportunities promoted by the hospital administration.

HYGIENE

Hygiene is the science of health and its preservation. The term also refers to practices that are conductive to good health. Good personal hygiene usually means those measures a person takes to keep his skin and its appendages (his hair, finger nails, and toe nails) and his health & mouth clean and in good condition. Physical health is an important component of total health. The subject of physical health includes care of the skin, hair, teeth, eyes, ears, hands, feet, rest & sleep, exercise, recreation & posture. The students must know not only the anatomy of the body organs but also known how these can be maintained in a state of optimum health. The science of preserving and promoting health is known as hygiene. Hygiene has two aspects:

- Personal Hygiene
- Environmental Hygiene

The Subject of personal hygiene is physical health and how to maintain it. Preventive medicine is defined as "The Science and art of preventing decease, prolonging life & promoting physical and mental health and efficiency". Where as in preventive medicine the focus is on the individual in community health. Personal Hygiene helps in the following manner:

- To maintain a good and clean physique.
- To maintain good muscle strength.
- To maintain clean mouth and Teeth free from carries.

- To keep the eyes, ears and nose in a healthy condition and free from infection.
- To maintain a healthy skin.
- To preserve ones energy and not get tired in carrying out daily tasks.
- To maintain resistance and prevent infection.

HYGIENE PRINCIPLES

- The intact skin is the body first organ of defence against infection and injury.
- Individual differences exit in the nature of the skin and its appendages.
- Changes occur throughout the life span in the skin, mucus membrane, hair, nails and the teeth.
- The health of the skin and mucus membrane is highly dependant on adequate nourishment, fluid intake and exercise.
- A person general health affects both the status of his skin and appendages, teeth and mouth.
- Hygiene practices are learnt.
- Hygiene practices vary with cultural norms, personal values and ability to maintain good habits of cleanliness and grooming.
- Drugs and other form of therapeutic treatment affect the skin and its appendages.

NURSING

Most people think of Nursing as caring for the sick or helping the doctor in the care and treatment of patients. It is much more than this, nursing includes carrying activities in hospital and in community. Nursing includes preventing illness, disability and death. Nursing responsibility is also includes health education, research, training and supervision of health personnel and administration.

Nursing is helping a person with those things he cannot do for himself, but are necessary for him to get back to his former health and independence. In nursing we should try to do even more. We should do, all we can to help people to live a life that is fully healthy in body, mind and spirit and social relationship. When nursing an individual we should remember his feelings and beliefs, try to understand his problems, also the needs of his family and of the community. Nursing is an important part of work of a health worker.

PERSONAL HYGIENE

Skin Care

To preserve cleanliness of skin and to keep healthy, regular baths and proper clothing are necessary. Other wise, the sebaceous glands will be locked, which in turn will interfere with the excretion process and further lead to certain skin condition such as scabies, impetigo, prickly heat and ring worm etc. Skin is the one of the most vital organ of the body. The functions of the skin are:

- It protects the body from heat, cold, humidity and entry of micro organisms.
- It acts as a sensory agent for touch.
- It converts sunlight into vitamin D.

Bathing of the skin: Skin comes in contact with the external environment and accumulates dirt. Taking daily bath with soap and water removes dirt and free us from all body odours. Soap is good surface cleaning agent. It gives a sense of freshness and well being and also prevents infection. Bathing help not only in cleanliness, but also in maintaining good circulation of blood, tone of muscle and improves appetite. Baths may vary according to climatic conditions and be classified according to condition of the patient and temperature of the water. Main purposes of bath are: -

- To remove waste products and clean the skin.
- To refresh and promote relaxation.
- To stimulate circulation.
- To maintain the condition of the skin.
- The best time for the bath is either before breakfast or at least one hour after meals.

The skin must be maintain and protected by the following ways:

Regular baths: A daily bath, taken twice a day, is essential in India because of the hot climate. It keeps the skin clean and prevents infections such as boils, scabies, ringworm and itching.

Oil baths: Periodical oil baths are beneficial especially during winter months for healthy skin and prevention of dryness of the skin.

Balanced diet: A daily balanced diet and a diet including vitamin A rich foods should be taken to promote health of the skin.

Mosquito nets: The skin is a portal of entry to many communicable diseases such as malaria and filariasis through insect bites. So the people must use mosquito nets to prevent insect bites.

Protective clothing: People who are working in industries and factories, those who come in contact with acids, alkalis and other chemical and physical agents should wear protective cloths to prevent accidents and injuries.

Cosmetics: As long as there is no allergy and skin irritation, they should be no objection in using cosmetics. Overuse of cosmetics may cause more harm than benefits because this may blocks the sweat glands.

Clothing: Clothing is one of the essential needs of the man. The main purposes of clothing are:

- To protect the body from climatic factors such as extreme cold and heat, to protect from injuries and bites of animals and insects.
- To maintain the body heat.
- For personal value such as ornamentation and decoration.

Choice of clothing is important and the material for clothing should be appropriate, for example, wool is best clothing for winter season. Cotton cloths are best in summer season. So, one should wear clean cloths after bath.

Hair Care

The condition of hair often reflects the general condition of the body and its nutritional status. In children who have streaked, yellowish brown, dry hair indicates deficiency of vitamins. In kwashiorkor hair becomes thin, sparse and easily breakable. Hair breaking shows that the shafts are not receiving sufficient nourishment. Greying or loss of hair pigment is due to deficiency of diet, physical and mental diseases. Using of soaps, shampoos and soap nuts take care of the hair. Soaps are mostly made up of with animal or vegetable oil such as coconut oil, olive oil, glycerine and sandalwood.

A good shampoo is prepared from synthetic detergents and it removes the surface grease, dirt and skin debris without affecting the scalp. Soap nuts are natural products and cause no harm to hair and remove dirt thoroughly. After using these, we should wash hair thoroughly with warm water. Before and during washing, the scalp should be massaged properly with the fingertips. The regular care of the hair is washing with shampoo, twice a week. Massaging the scalp is also useful. It is a type of positive exercise. It stimulates the blood flow and improves the nutrition of the hair. Oils are easily absorbed in the skin. So, once in a week massaging the scalp with coconut oil is very beneficial. Good scalp hygiene prevents infections like scabies, head lice, ringworm and dandruff.

Dandruff: Dandruff is due to the excessive shedding of dead skin cells from the scalp. As it is normal for skin cells to die and flake off, a small amount of flaking is normal and in fact quite common. Some people, however, either chronically or as a result of certain triggers, experience an unusually large amount of flaking, which can also be accompanied by redness and irritation. Most cases of dandruff can be easily treated with specialized shampoos. Excessive flaking can also be a symptom of seborrhoeic dermatitis, psoriasis, fungal infection or excoriation associated with infestation of head lice.

Those affected by dandruff find that it can cause social or self-esteem problems. Treatment may be important purely for psychological reasons. Regular washing with shampoo can control dandruff. Shampoo containing selenium and sulphur are available in the market to treat dandruff, but they should not be use regularly.

Pediculosis: For infestation of lice or pediculosis, one part of kerosene, one part of the pure oil may be rubbed well into the hair at night, covered with a towel or a cap, and the hair washed next morning. Warm vinegar will soften the nits and then they can be washed off the hair. The more recent treatment is 10% DDT dusting powder applied to the hair and covered with a towel for several hours. The hair can be combed with a fine toothcomb and DDT applied again a week later. In the meantime the hair should not be washed after the first dusting so that the new lice can be killed as they hatch.

Oral Hygiene

The care of the teeth is explained below:

Tooth brushing: Teeth should be cleaned at least twice a day. Many people in the village use tender twigs of neem or babbul (acacia) as a toothbrush. Some use ash, charcoal and some tooth powders. The toothbrush is the best for removal of food debris and dental plaque, which accumulates around the neck of the teeth. Along with the toothpaste and powders, tooth brushing is ideal for cleaning the teeth. The bristles of the toothbrush should be soft that and should not be too sharp or too hard.

For brushing the teeth generally a vertical or circular brushing techniques are recommended. Tooth should be clean and the mouth should be rinsed soon after eating food. The tongue should be scraped or brushed and the mouth should be gargled with luke-warm water to keep the throat clean.

Use of fluorides: Where ever drinking water contains less than 0.5 mg of fluorides per litre, excessive dental caries has been observed. The optimum level of fluoride in drinking water is between 0.5 to 0.8 mg per litre. Fluorides decreases enamel solubility in acids. Deficiency of fluorine in drinking water can be rectified by applying topical fluoride on the tooth surfaces. The use of fluorides is significant means of caries prevention. Fluoride present in the drinking water acts both systemically and locally.

Regular Dental checkups: Dental check-up twice a year is recommended for early diagnosis and treatment of dental ailments. In some countries, regular dental services or check ups are provided to all school children through school dental nurses and dental hygienists.

Diet: The relation between the diet and dental disease is well known. In cities the dental disease are increased. Excessive intake of refined carbohydrates such as sugar sweets, jilebees, pastries, cakes, chocolates and biscuits promotes the dental caries. Soft and sticky foods that adhere to the teeth causes tooth decay. Intake of fruits, vegetables like carrots, cucumber, sugarcane etc. reduces the frequency of dental caries. These foods are called natural toothbrushes and their daily intake should be promoted.

Habits: The habit of sucking sweets in the mouth causes a marked increased in tooth decay. Holding a feeding bottle with milk or sweetened juices for a long time sucking may cause dental caries. This is called by dentists "baby bottle syndrome". The habit of eating snacks frequently in between meals is also a bad habit. The habit of chewing betel leaves and tobacco is an important cause of bad oral hygiene in India. The foundation of good oral hygiene is laid in early childhood.

Care of dentures: Dentures are man-made substitutes. All dentures are potentially traumatic. These should be removed after meals and thoroughly brushed. All dentures must be removed at night because they can act as incubators of bacteria. After removing the dentures the mouth should be rinsed thoroughly with warm salt water. Don't place the dentures in boiling water. Dentures can be washed with baking soda or any washing detergent.

Care of the Hands and Nails

Hands and nails are never free from micro organisms. They pick up dirt and bacteria easily because they come in contact with many things. Therefore they should be kept clean, by thoroughly washing with soap and water, especially before taking food. After attending the toilet, hands should be washed with soap and water. The nails collect dirt, so they should be kept clean by gentle scrubbing with nailbrush. The habit of biting nails and putting fingers in the nose or ears and mouth is unhygienic habit and this should be discouraged.

Nails also require rigorous cleaning. They need to be cut short periodically. Otherwise dirt will be accumulate under long nails which is unhygienic, harbour harmful organisms of typhoid, cholera, dysentery, diarrhoea and various intestinal worms. Long nails can also be dangerous like scratching or hurting the skin of a patient while giving care, especially in cases of newborn and children.

Hand washing: In the community health nursing practice, if a nurse has to wash hands before carrying out any procedure, following technique can be followed, that is wet the hands from elbow towards fingertips and apply soap well. Rub the hands thoroughly and washed the tips of fingers and thumb in and out, then wash between fingers and arms rotating motion, a rinse from elbow to the downward this helps to remove dirt. Repeat it whenever necessary to remove adhered dirt.

Care of the Elimination

The organs of elimination are the lungs, skin, kidney and the intestine. These are involuntary acts. The elimination of faeces is a voluntary action. Lungs eliminate carbon dioxide, skin eliminates sweat, and kidneys eliminate urine.

Kidney: Proper maintenance of skin as mentioned earlier and good exercise will promote elimination of wastes thoroughly by kidneys. The kidneys excrete 3-4 pints of water per a day.

Bowel: Forming a regular habit of emptying the bowels each day at about the same time will help in avoiding constipation. Some guidance and a bit of permissiveness will help the child to establish his own schedule. Irregularity of bowel habits may cause the individual to have headaches, be impatient, low spirited, or lack of energy and will be unable to concentrate and study. The hands need to be washed well with soap and water afterwards. Open field defecation is to be avoided.

Menstrual Hygiene

The menstruating woman is considered unclean and is prevented from taking part in normal daily activities in some communities. It should be explained that menstruation is a normal physiological process. The menstrual discharge is usually controlled by means of an absorbent sanitary pad or diaper, which must be frequently changed. Alternatively an absorbent tampon may be placed in the vagina.

Intra-vaginal tampons fitted with a cord are available. Commercially they are easy to insert and remove. Intra-vaginal tampons are popular because they are comfortable and convenient. Their main disadvantage is that they cannot be used unless the hymen is torn or stretched. Vaginal douching is not only unnecessary at the end of the period or at any other time, but is positively harmful in that it washes away the natural protective discharge. The vagina can take care of it self, and it is remarkable how it cleanses itself of all the menstrual debris in the course of a few hours. Regarding sexual intercourse during menstruation, there is no medical reason to avoid, but only objection is the obvious aesthetic one.

Eye Care

Eye often reflects the physical health. Eyes needs well maintained care. When reading books they should be held 12 to 16 inches away from the eye at an angle of 45° to 75°. Skin around eyes must be cleaned with soap and water or clear water. Vitamin A foods are used for good eyesight and prevent infractions.The conditions which may affect the eyes are:

- Infections-conjunctivitis, trachoma, sty
- Injuries-corneal ulcers
- Malnutrition-Night blindness, exophthalmia
- Errors of refraction - short sightedness, long-sightedness.
- Others- cataract, glaucoma.

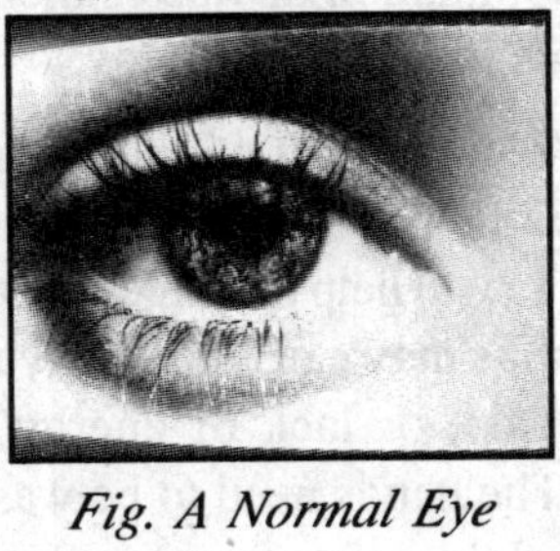

Fig. A Normal Eye

There are 15 million blind people in India as of year 2007. The main causes of blindness are:

- Cataract.
- Trachoma.
- Others infections.
- Malnutrition.
- Injuries.
- Glaucoma.

Blindness is preventable through simple measures such as:

- Early diagnosis and treatment
- Good personal hygiene.
- Improvement in diet.
- Control of flies.
- Health education.

The care of the eyes consists of the following:

- Prevention and control of infections.
- Injuries.
- Eye strain
- Good diet.
- Squint
- Regular check up

Prevention and Control of Infections: Eye is a delicate and sensitive organ. Trachoma is eye infection which is common in children. It spread by using infected clothes, handkerchiefs, towels, and flies. Conjunctivitis is an acute inflammation of the outer layers of the eye which is caused by bacteria, virus or allergy. The preventive measures are:

- Early diagnosis and treatment until cure is achieved
- Health education towards of clean towels and linen, fly control, prevention and good personal hygiene.

Injuries: During working or playing, eye is exposed to injuries. In industries, eye injuries are common; workers must use protective glasses. In children eye injuries are due to firecrackers. While playing they may cause eye injury. Foreign bodies also cause eye injury. Wash the eye immediately with plenty of water, eye should not be rubbed. If foreign body does not come out, refer to doctor immediately.

Eye Strain: Reading must be done in good light to avoid eyestrain. Light should come from left and behind. Hold the book at 45 to 75 degrees from the horizontal level. Avoid reading in moving trains and buses or in lying positions. Eye must be protected from direct exposure to sun light, glare and extreme brightness. If required wear glasses.

Good diet: Many eye diseases occur due to malnutrition. Vitamin A rich foods such as green leafy vegetables, fruits, milk and butter prevent deficiency diseases like neurosis, keratomalaia, night blindness.

Squint: If there is a cross eye or squint, refer to specialist. This defect can be rectified by the use of glasses or eye exercises. In some cases, it may need operation. It should be treated early in the life.

Regular check-up: Regular check up by the eye specialist once a year until the age of 10 and there after every 3 years is must in early detection and treatment of eye diseases.

Care of the Ears

The ear is an important sense organ of the body. It is useful not only for hearing, but also for body equilibrium. The ear is liable to infection and injury. Infections of nose and throat readily spread to middle ear and cause inflammation known as otitis media. The ear problems are earache, discharge, wax and foreign bodies.

Care of the ear comprises of the following:

- Keeping the ear clean.
- Removing excessive wax carefully
- Preventing entering of water into the ear during bathing.
- Protect the ear from exposure to loud noises.
- Preventing and treating all nose and throat infections.
- If the ear canal is full of wax it must be cleaned. For its removal, put a drop of warm boiled coconut oil, olive oil, peanut oil or glycerine into the ear.
- Teaching good habits; one should not put pencils, patches and other foreign bodies into ear. If any foreign body enter into the ear refer to a doctor.

Care of Nose and Throat

Great care should be taken in blowing the nose. If possible, have disposable tissues for nasal discharge or cough. If not, rag pieces may be used (placed in covered vessel of water after use and boiled for 10 minutes then washed and hung in the sun to dry). Sari ends or fingers should never be used. When swimming keep water as much as out of the nose and throat and be sure the water is safe, (not contaminated) by waste materials. While the face is under water, expel air slowly and continuously through the nose. Breathe in through the mouth while the head is above water. Blow the nose gently after swimming. If there is any infection of nose or throat, it may spread rapidly to ear. Treat the infection immediately.

Care of the Feet

The human foot is composed of 26 bones, connected by ligaments, muscles, blood vessels and nerves. Bones are so arranged as to balance and support the weight of the body. If the foot are allowed to stay in a wrong position for a long time, it leads to poor posture. To prevent diseases and for foot hygiene, the feet should be washed with soap and water, both at night and morning. The feet may be soaked in a dilute solution of formalin (table spoon of formalin to 250 ml. of water) for 15 minutes, then thoroughly dried and dusted with boric acid or talcum powder. Special care must be taken in selection of shoes. Shoes must be broad-toed and not too fitting. The socks should be clean and dry and they should not be too tight. Walking bare foot is unhygienic. Avoid cuts and bruises. If occurs, they should be treated with mild antiseptic cream. If there are cracks, apply milk cream or coconut oil.

PATIENT ENVIRONMENT

The environment is an important element in the care that patients receive. Visitors, carers and staff are also concerned with the environment especially if it is inadequate or dirty. Areas covered are under patient environment are:

- Clean hospitals.
- Hospital food.
- Ward Housekeeping.
- Patient environment networks.
- Privacy and dignity.

PATIENT BEDS

Providing a clean, comfortable bed and positioning a patient in the optimum posture for prevention of complications and to enable maximum independence are fundamental nursing skills. Bed making is a daily routine that requires practical and technical skills. Selecting the correct posture for a patient in bed or in a chair is essential for physiological functioning and recovery. In this article bed making is described, as are positioning and re-positioning in relation to patients in bed, armchairs and wheelchairs. Infection control and moving and handling issues are also considered.

Guidelines for Bed-making

Gather all the needed linen and accessories before making the bed.

- Sheets.
- Pillowcases.
- Blankets.
- Bedspread.
- Extra pillows.

Avoid shaking the linen to prevent the spread of micro organisms and dust particles.

Avoid placing linens, clean or dirty, on another patient's bed.

Do not place dirty linen on the floor.

Do not hold dirty linen against your uniform.

Always use good body mechanics; raise the bed to its highest position to make bed-making easier.

Stay on one side of the bed until it is completely made; then move to the other side and finish the bed. This saves time and steps.

Observe the patient and document any nursing observations.

- Check for areas of redness that may lead to decubiti formation.
- Note tolerance of activity level while out of bed.
- Note observations about the physical and emotional status of the patient.
- Note any patient teaching or reinforced teaching given and the patient's response.
- Check for drainage, wetness, or other body fluids and record observations.

TYPES OF BEDS

Unoccupied (Closed) Bed

An unoccupied bed is one that is made when not occupied by a patient:

- Raise the bed to a comfortable working height, if adjustable.
- Lower side-rails, if present.
- Remove pillows and pillowcases. Set the pillows aside in a clean area.
- Fold and set the blankets and spreads aside (to be reused).
- Loosen the linen along the edges of the bed, and move toward the end of the bed.
- Wash the mattress if necessary, turn the mattress to the opposite side if necessary, and replace the mattress pad as required. Observe the mattress for protruding springs.
- Place the bottom sheet.

Flat Sheet

- Position evenly on the bed.
- Miter the corners at the top of the bed. Lift the mattress slightly, then stretch and tie the ends of the sheet together beneath the mattress. Repeat these steps for the bottom of the bed.
- Stretch and tuck the free edges at the sides.

Fitted Sheet

1. Fit the sheet on the lower edges of the mattress first. Then lift the mattress and fit the sheet on the top edges of the mattress.
2. Stretch and tuck the free edges at the sides.
3. Place a draw sheet on the centre of the bed, if it is required.
    - Tuck in the free edge on one side.
    - Stretch the draw sheet from the opposite side and tuck in the free edge.
4. Place the top sheet, blanket (if used), and bedspread.
    - Position evenly on the bed.
    - Miter the bottom corners, tucking all three parts together.
    - Leave the loose ends free.
5. Fanfold the top linen back to the foot of the bed.
6. Place a clean pillowcase over the pillow and place it at the head of the bed.
    - Invert the pillowcase over one hand so the inner back seam is visible.

- Grasp the edge of the pillow with one hand holding the pillowcase at the seam.
- Use the opposite hand to guide the pillowcase over the pillow.

7. Adjust the bed to its lowest position, if adjustable.
8. Reposition the head up slightly, if the patient prefers.
9. Raise the side-rail opposite the side of the bed where the patient will enter.

Occupied (Open) Bed

An occupied bed is one that is made while occupied by a patient:

1. Wash your hands.
2. Identify the patient, explain the procedure, and be sure you will have the patient's cooperation.
3. Check the condition of the bed linens to determine which supplies you will need.
4. Provide for the patient's privacy (throughout the procedure).
5. Obtain the articles of linen that you will need.
6. Place the bath blanket over the patient and the top cover.
7. Loosen the top bedding from the foot of the bed and remove it. If possible, have the patient hold the bath blanket while you pull the top covers from under it from the foot of the bed.
8. Move the mattress to the head of the bed.
9. Move the patient to the distal side of the bed.
10. Make the bed on one side.
11. Move or turn the patient to the clean side of the bed, and finish making the bed on the opposite side. Place the clean linen on top, and remove the bath blanket.
12. Attach the patient's signal cord within reach.
13. Provide for the patient's safety and comfort.
14. Tidy the room.

PHYSIOLOGICAL NEEDS

Patients who have emerged from low awareness states may present with psychological needs that can be addressed via adapted formal clinical psychological interventions, or by behavioural techniques. Families of these patients may experience similar psychological reactions to relatives of any patients with severe brain injury, but there are also additional components that are unique to patients in low awareness states.

These sources of psychological distress for relatives are discussed. The needs of clinicians working with these clients are also discussed. It is significant that services attending to the needs of clients in low awareness states also have adequate support for both relatives and clinicians.

Understanding a person's physiological and psychological needs is essential for every health care worker. Every individual has needs that must be satisfied to maintain stability. Health care workers must be aware of these needs to maintain their own stability and to meet the needs of patients and co-workers.

Biological needs are the fundamental needs for survival. They include food, water, sleep, and elimination. Any one or several of these needs may be threatened by illness. Food and water are often withheld prior to surgery or other procedures. Sleep may be interrupted by the change of environment, unfamiliar noises, or anxiety when hospitalization is required. Elimination is frequently affected by a change in routine, foods, or medications. Though these changes are temporary, they do affect patients.

Communications explains to new patients about mealtimes, how to request water or snacks, and any special orders for using the bathroom. Always explain expected interruptions in routine as soon as possible. When sleep must be interrupted, inform the patient before he or she goes to sleep. It is significant to adapt the way you communicate this information to patients in accordance with their age or level of understanding. Show your commitment to treating others with dignity by using effective communication skills. Communicating to patients how their biological needs will be met during their hospitalization helps eradicate fear and anxiety.

Safety needs are the need to feel secure and the need to avoid bodily harm ad injury. When patients are ill, they may feel very insecure and frightened. They may be facing outpatient procedures they do not understand, such as injections or therapies that are frightening to them. They may be facing hospitalization for the first time and are afraid that they will be hurt or that they will die. Geriatric clients have these fears, also. They may be entering a nursing home where they will stay for the rest of their lives. They wonder, What will happen to me? How will I be treated? Will I be safe?

SLEEP AND REST

THE PHYSIOLOGY OF SLEEP

Sleep is a part of the daily routine in everyone, even when the "normal" sleep/wake pattern is disrupted by outside components. In this section we will use the "normal" circadian rhythm (from the Latin words circa "about" and dies "the day") of day/night activities to explore the chemistry and physiology of sleep. In humans, the circadian cycle operates in a 24 to 25 hour cycle measured from awakening after one sleep period to awakening from the next sleep period.

The physiologic mechanisms of circadian rhythm begin when light strikes special cells within the retina of the eye which, in turn, causes these cells to secrete a special hormone that causes an area of the brain known as the suprachiasmatic nucleus to signal the pineal body to stop secreting the hormone melatonin, which has been shown to reach its highest levels during sleep. As the day progresses, a chemical called adenosine accumulates within the brain as the level of melatonin falls.

As night falls the inhibitory effects of the retinal secretions on the pineal body are removed allows the pineal to begin secreting melatonin once again. It is the presence of higher melatonin levels within certain areas of the brain (such as the thalamus and hypothalamus) that controls the urge to sleep.

FACTORS AFFECTING SLEEP

Depressants

Tryptophan: The amino acid tryptophan is a building block of the protein found in foods. It contributes to sleepiness. Carbohydrates make tryptophan more available to the brain, which is why carbohydrate-heavy meals containing tryptophan tend to cause drowsiness. Tryptophan is a precursor to the neurotransmitter serotonin, which is a precursor to the neurohormone melatonin.

Melatonin: Melatonin is a naturally occurring hormone that regulates sleepiness. It is made in the brain where tryptophan is converted into serotonin and then into melatonin, which is released at night by the pineal gland to induce and maintain sleep. Melatonin supplementation may be used as a sleep aid, both as a hypnotic and as a chronobiotic.

The "Post-Lunch Dip": Many people have a temporary drop in alertness in early afternoon, usually known as the post-lunch dip. While a large meal, rich in carbohydrates, can make an individual feel sleepy, the post-lunch dip is mostly an effect of the biological clock. People naturally feel most sleepy (have the greatest "drive for sleep") at two times of the day about 12 hours apart, for instance at 2: 00 AM and 2: 00 PM. At those two times, the body clock "kicks in". At about 2 p.m. (14: 00), it overrides the homeostatic build-up of sleep debt, allowing several more hours of wakefulness. At about 2 a.m. (02: 00), with the daily sleep debt paid off, it "kicks in" again to ensure a few more hours of sleep.

Alcohol: Often people start drinking alcohol in order to get to sleep (alcohol is initially a sedative and will make you get to sleep faster). However, being addicted to alcohol can lead to disrupted sleep because alcohol has a rebound effect later in the night. As a result there is strong evidence linking alcoholism and insomnia.

Barbiturates: Barbiturates when taken cause drowsiness and have actions similar to ethanol (drinking alcohol).

Anti-Depressants

Caffeine: Caffeine is a stimulant that works by slowing the action of the hormones in the brain that cause sleepiness. Effective dosage is individual, in part dependent on prior usage. It can cause a rapid reduction in alertness as it wears off.

Energy Drinks: The stimulating effects of energy drinks comes from natural stimulants such as caffeine, sugars, and essential amino acids, and eventually will create a rapid reduction in alertness similar to that of caffeine.

Amphetamines: Amphetamines (amphetamine, dextroamphetamine, methamphetamine, etc) are often used to treat narcolepsy and ADHD disorders. The most common effects are decreased appetite, stimulation and insomnia, and increased alertness.

Cocaine and Crack Cocaine: Similar in action to the amphetamines.

MDMA: Usually known as ecstasy, users are kept awake similar to amphetamines with intense euphoria, includes other similar drugs like MDA, MMDA, or bk-MDMA.

Methylphenidate: Usually known as Ritalin, similar in action to amphetamines and cocaine.

PROMOTING REST AND SLEEP

Promoting an environment conducive to sleep in hospital is a challenge. Though patients may appear to sleep in hospital, it may not be refreshing or restorative. The reasons for this can be categorized into three groups: environmental, physiological and psychological. These components can work concomitantly, making sleep virtually impossible for some patients. Nurses can help their patients by understanding what influences sleep patterns and acting on this knowledge. This may include a variety of interventions, from allowing patients to carry out their own bedtime routine, to explaining to elderly people how their sleeping patterns change with age.

SLEEP DISORDERS

A sleep disorder is loosely defined as any condition or process that alters the patient's previously established sleep/wake cycle. As with many other medical conditions, sleep disorders span a spectrum that ranges from inconvenience to potentially life threatening. Sleep disorders are divided into two general classes: Dysomnias and Parasomnias.

Dysomnias are conditions that manifest themselves as either hypersomnia (abnormal sleep cycles causing the urge to sleep at times when the circadian cycle would suggest that wakefulness was appropriate) or insomnia (the inability to sleep). The dysomnias can be further subdivided into three classes that are dependent on the source of the sleep interference:

Intrinsic (arising within the body): Primary insomnia, obstructive sleep apnea, restless leg disorder, and unspecified limb movements

Extrinsic (arising outside the body): Environmental conditions not conducive to uninterrupted sleep such as noise of ambient temperature.

Alteration or interference with the circadian rhythm: Jet lag or variations in occupational schedules (shift work).

Parasomnias include sleep terror (sudden awakening and unreasonable fear), bedwetting, somnambulism (sleep walking), and somniloquy (talking in one's sleep).

NUTRITION

Nutrition (also called nourishment or aliment) is the provision, to cells and organisms, of the materials necessary (in the form of food) to support life. Many common health problems can be prevented or alleviated with good nutrition.

The diet of an organism refers to what it eats. Dieticians are health professionals who specialize in human nutrition, meal planning, economics, preparation, and so on. They are trained to provide safe, evidence-based dietary advice and management to persons (in health and disease), as well as to institutions. Poor diet can have an injurious impact on health, causing deficiency diseases such as scurvy, beriberi, and kwashiorkor; health-threatening conditions like obesity and metabolic syndrome, and such common chronic systemic diseases as cardiovascular disease, diabetes, and osteoporosis.

IMPORTANCE

Good nutrition is significant for everyone. Healthful diets help children grow, develop, and do well in school. They enable people of all ages to work productively and feel their best. What people eat can also help reduce the risk for chronic diseases, such as heart disease, certain cancers, diabetes, stroke, and osteoporosis, which are foremost causes of death and disability. Finally, eating right can reduce the risk of obesity, high blood pressure, and high blood cholesterol, which increase the risk of disease.

Proper nutrition means getting both enough calories and the proper nutrients. Many people in this country eat more calories than the body needs. This can lead to obesity which is a risk component for many diseases, like diabetes, heart disease, and cancer. It is significant to remember that, though an overweight individual may be getting more calories than required, he or she may not be getting all of the necessary nutrients.

Eating a daily diet that includes adequate amounts of bread, cereal, grain, rice, pasta, vegetables, and fruit, and limits high fat foods, can promote health and reduce the risk of developing certain chronic diseases.

FACTORS AFFECTING NUTRITIONAL NEEDS

Age: Growing ages can change the nutritional needs of a human being.

Diseases: Diseases also can change the nutritional needs of a man.

Pregnancy: Pregnancy in women can change the nutritional needs of a female.

Assessment of Nutritional Needs: Variables

Evaluating nutritional status achieves the following:

- Identifies actual nutritional deficiencies.
- Illuminates dietary patterns that may contribute to health problems.

- Provides a basis for planning for more optimal nutrition.
- Establishes baseline data for assessment.

One of the first steps in evaluating nutrition is screening the patient for possible nutritional risks. At the very least, you should evaluate the health history for symptoms and situations related to nutritional problems, perform a fundamental physical examination, and obtain laboratory data associated with malnutrition. A comprehensive nutritional evaluation involves a detailed dietary history, focused anthropometry, and assessment of laboratory values. It is recommended for people with any of the following nutritional risks:

- Weight less than 80 percent or more than 120 percent of ideal body weight (IBW).
- History of unintentional weight loss (10 lb or 10 percent of usual weight).
- Serum albumin concentration lower than 3.5 g/dL.
- Total lymphocyte count lower than 1500 cells/mm3.
- History of illness, surgery, trauma, or stress.
- Symptoms associated with nutritional deficiency or depletion.
- Factors associated with inadequate nutritional intake or absorption.

MEETING NUTRITIONAL NEEDS

Nutrients are substances contained in food that are essential for optimal body functioning. The primary nutrients are carbohydrates, proteins, fats, vitamins, minerals, and water. Carbohydrates, protein, and fat are the body's major energy sources. Carbohydrates and protein each supply 4 calories per gram, and fat provides 9 calories per gram. Vitamins are essential to specific functions in the body. Minerals are inorganic elements that are essential to cell structure and physiological functions in the body. Water makes up 50 to 60 percent of the adult weight. It is needed for many functions, and humans cannot survive for more than a few days without it.

Vegetarian Diets

Fats: Lipids or fats are insoluble in water and soluble in alcohol, ether, and chloroform. They include true fats, lipids, Vegetarian diets consist primarily of plant foods. Vegans avoid all animal products in the diet, lactovegetarians eat dairy products, and lacto-ovovegetarians also eat eggs. Though these diets provide less protein than nonvegetarian diets, they meet or exceed the RDAs. Whole grains, legumes, vegetables, seeds, and nuts contain all the essential and nonessential amino acids. As long as food intake is varied and calories are sufficient, protein deficiencies will not occur. Furthermore, soy protein provides all essential and nonessential amino acids and is nutritionally equivalent to animal sources of protein. It can serve as the sole source of protein if desired. However, because significant variation exists, evaluate the adequacy of vegetarian diets on an individual basis.

Highly saturated fat (solid at room temperature) significantly contributes to elevated serum triglyceride and cholesterol levels. Unsaturated and polyunsaturated fats are recommended because of their inverse relationship with heart disease.

Cholesterol occurs naturally and exclusively in all animal food products. The body needs cholesterol for cell structure, as a precursor for certain hormones and vitamins, and to aid in the digestive process. But even if no cholesterol were consumed in the diet, the body would synthesize the required supply. Serum cholesterol and lipids attach to proteins and are transported throughout the body as lipoproteins.

Vitamins are organic compounds that play a major role in enzyme reactions associated with the metabolism of carbohydrate, protein, and fat. Though vitamins are needed in small amounts, the body does not synthesize them, so they must be present in the diet.

Minerals are inorganic compounds found in nature. They play a wide variety of roles in human nutrition.

Minerals are needed in varying amounts and are divided into major and trace elements.

Water helps regulate body temperature; serves as a solvent for vitamins, minerals, and other nutrients; acts as a medium for chemical reactions; serves as a lubricant; and transports nutrients to and wastes from the cells.

URINARY ELIMINATION

Elimination of urine is an essential bodily function, but independence in this activity may be affected by physical and mental disability. Part 1 of this article discusses the anatomy and physiology of the renal and urinary tract and the production of urine. Urinalysis is a vital nursing evaluation and the collection of specimens and the range of tests undertaken are outlined. Assisting patients to use the toilet, commode or bedpan is an essential nursing skill. The significance of sensitivity, empathy and moving and handling risk evaluation is discussed, and the evaluation and management of urinary tract infection and urinary tract stones are addressed.

PHYSIOLOGY OF URINE ELIMINATION

Urinary tract is divided into four parts:

Kidneys

- Two reddish-brown, bean-shaped organs located on either side of the vertebral column behind the abdominal peritoneum and against the deep muscles of the back
- Each kidney has its own blood supply
- One renal artery
  1. Originates in the abdominal aorta
  2. Enters the kidney at the hilum
- One renal vein
  1. Exits the kidney through the hilum
  2. Joins the inferior vena cava
- Each kidney has over 1,000,000 nephrons, its functional unit that filters waste products from the blood and regulates fluid and electrolyte concentrations in the body fluids, which are composed of six parts
  1. Glomerulus
  2. Bowman's capsule
  3. Proximal convoluted tubule
  4. Loop of Henle
  5. Distal convoluted tubule
  6. Collecting duct

Ureters

- Two tubular structures attached to each kidney pelvis which carry urine from the kidneys into the bladder
- Length of the ureters
- 25 to 30 centimetres (10 to 12 inches) long
- A small, flaplike fold of mucous membrane covers the junction of the ureters and the bladder and acts as a valve to prevent urinary reflux (backflow)

Bladder

- A hollow, distensible, muscular organ that is a reservoir for urine
- Composed of three parts
    - Detrusor muscle
        - Composed of three layers of smooth muscle
        - Inner; longitudinal
        - Middle; circular
        - Outer; longitudinal
    - The trigone (a triangle-shaped area located at the base of the bladder)
    - The ureter openings at the posterior corners form the base of the triangle
    - The opening of the urethra at the anterior inferior corner forms the apex of the triangle
    - Internal urinary sphincter (involuntary control; sits at the base of the bladder)

Urethra

- A tubular structure attached to the bladder that carries urine from the bladder to the urinary meatus and outside of the body
- Length of the urethra
- Women: 3.7 centimetres (1.5 inches) long
- Men: 20 centimetres (8 inches) long
- Comprises of three parts
    - Prostatic
    - Membranous
    - Cavernous
- Significant in renal and reproductive functioning
- Carries urine outside the body
- Carries semen outside the body
- External urinary sphincter (voluntary control) sits at the base of the urethra

CHARACTERISTICS OF URINE

Normal

- Amount (in 24 hours for adults): 1200 - 1500
- Colour: straw, amber, transparent

- Clarity: clear liquid
- Odour: faint aromatic
- Sterility: no micro organisms present
- pH: 4.5 to 8
- Specific gravity: 1.010 - 1.025
- Glucose: not present
- Ketone bodies: not present
- Blood: not present

Abnormal

- Amount (in 24 hours for adults): under 1200 or over 1500
- Colour: dark amber, cloudy, dark orange, red, dark brown
- Clarity: mucus plugs, viscid, thick
- Odour: offensive
- Sterility: micro organisms present
- pH: under 4.5 or over 8
- Specific gravity: under 1.010 or over 1.025
- Glucose: present
- Ketone bodies: present
- Blood: occult, bright red

ALTERATIONS IN URINARY ELIMINATION

Urinary incontinence and urinary retention are the most common causes of altered urinary elimination patterns. Urinary incontinence is the uncontrolled loss of urine that constitutes a social or hygienic problem. Urinary retention is the inability to completely evacuate urine from the bladder during micturition.

There are two primary types of urinary incontinence, acute and chronic. In addition, chronic urinary incontinence can be subdivided into several distinctive types. Because each has its own etiology and management, it is important to determine the type of incontinence before subjecting the client to the expense, potential risks, and rigors of a treatment program.

Acute Urinary Incontinence

Acute urinary incontinence is a transient and reversible loss of urine. It may occur during an acute illness or after an injury. Common causes of acute urinary incontinence include urinary tract infection, atrophic vaginitis, polyuria related to diabetes, acute confusion, immobility, and sedation. Medications that increase or decrease bladder or urethral sphincter tone also may contribute to acute incontinence.

Chronic Urinary Incontinence

Acute incontinence is distinguished from established or chronic incontinence. There are four predominant types of chronic urine loss:

- Stress urinary incontinence
- Instability incontinence
- Functional incontinence
- Extraurethral incontinence

Stress Urinary Incontinence: Stress urinary incontinence (SUI) is the uncontrolled loss of urine caused by physical exertion in the absence of a detrusor muscle contraction. SUI is associated with urethral hypermobility or with intrinsic sphincter deficiency. Urethral hypermobility is the abnormal movement of the bladder base and urethra during physical exertion. The relationship between urethral hypermobility and SUI is not entirely understood, although several mechanisms have been proposed. Descent of the urethra into the lower portion of the pelvis may cause a loss of abdominal pressure transmission when compared with forces that affect the bladder. In addition, muscular contraction is compromised in the hypermobile urethra. Loss of the normal anatomical relationships between the urethral sphincter and related structures also may contribute to SUI by reducing the efficiency of the muscular elements of the sphincter.

The contribution of estrogen deficiency, which compromises the elements of urethral coaptation in the woman, remains unclear. Intrinsic sphincter deficiency is a disorder of the muscular components of the urethral sphincter. Sphincter closure is compromised, and urinary leakage is often severe. Severe urine loss caused by intrinsic sphincter deficiency is defined as Total Incontinence. Unlike urethral hypermobility, which is a women's health concern, intrinsic sphincter deficiency occurs in both genders and is related primarily to iatrogenic or neuropathic causes. It is important to note that intrinsic sphincter deficiency and urethral hypermobility frequently coexist in women.

Instability Incontinence: Instability incontinence is the loss of urine caused by a premature or hyperactive contraction of the detrusor. In the person with normal sensations of the lower urinary tract, these unstable detrusor contractions initially cause a precipitous desire to urinate, followed by urinary leakage unless the opportunity to toilet is immediately available. In those without sensations of bladder filling and impending urination, the contraction is followed by urinary incontinence that is often described as unpredictable.

Urinary Retention

Urinary retention is caused by two conditions: bladder outlet obstruction and deficient detrusor muscle contraction strength. Bladder outlet obstruction causes incomplete bladder evacuation by blocking the outflow of urine through the sphincter mechanism or the urethra. Deficient detrusor muscle contraction strength occurs when contractions are insufficient to maintain urethral opening long enough for complete emptying of the bladder's contents. Because the management of each condition is different, it is important to differentiate between these disorders during evaluation.

TYPES OF COLLECTION OF URINE SPECIMEN

The urine specimen collection is a procedure used to obtain a sample of urine from a patient for diagnostic tests.

Types of Collection

- Random Specimen: This is the specimen most usually sent to the laboratory for analysis, primarily because it is the easiest to obtain and is readily available. This specimen is commonly submitted for urinalysis and microscopic analysis, though it is not the specimen of choice for either of these tests. Random specimens can sometimes give an inaccurate view of a patient's health if the specimen is too diluted and analyte values are artificially lowered.
- First Morning Specimen: This is the specimen of choice for urinalysis and microscopic analysis, since the urine is generally more concentrated (due to the length of time the urine is allowed to remain in the bladder) and, hence, contains relatively higher levels of cellular elements and analytes such as protein, if present. Also called an 8-hour specimen, the first morning specimen is collected when the patient first wakes up in the morning, having emptied the bladder before going to sleep. Since the urine can be collected over any eight-hour period, collection is practical for patients who have atypical work/ sleep schedules. Proper collection practices and accurate recording of the collection time are significant criteria of a

first morning specimen. Note: Any urine that is voided from the bladder during the eight-hour collection period should be pooled and refrigerated, so that a true 8-hour specimen is obtained.

- Midstream Clean Catch Specimen: This is the preferred type of specimen for culture and sensitivity testing because of the reduced incidence of cellular and microbial contamination. Patients are needed to first cleanse the urethral area with a castile soap towelette. The patient should then void the first portion of the urine stream into the toilet. These first steps significantly reduce the opportunities for contaminants to enter into the urine stream. The urine midstream is then collected into a clean container (any excess urine should be voided into the toilet). This method of collection can be conducted at any time of day or night.
- Timed Collection Specimen: Among the most usually performed tests requiring timed specimens are those measuring creatinine, urine urea nitrogen, glucose, sodium, potassium, or analytes such as catecholamines and 17-hydroxysteroids that are affected by diurnal variations.
- A timed specimen is collected to measure the concentration of these substances in urine over a specified length of time, commonly 8 or 24 hours. In this collection method, the bladder is emptied prior to beginning the timed collection. Then, for the duration of the designated time period, all urine is collected and pooled into a collection container, with the final collection taking place at the very end of that period. The specimen should be refrigerated during the collection period, unless otherwise requested by the physician. Accurate timing is critical to the calculations that are conducted to determine analyte concentrations and ratios. Interpretations based on faulty calculations can result in improper diagnoses or medical treatment.
- Catheter Collection Specimen: This assisted procedure is conducted when a patient is bedridden or cannot urinate independently. The healthcare provider inserts a Foley catheter into the bladder through the urethra to collect the urine specimen. (Specimens may also be collected through an existing Foley catheter.) Specimens may be collected directly from a

Foley into an evacuated tube or transferred from a syringe into a tube or cup.

- Suprapubic Aspiration Specimen: This method is used when a bedridden patient cannot be catheterized or a sterile specimen is needed. The urine specimen is collected by needle aspiration through the abdominal wall into the bladder.
- Paediatric Specimen: For infants and small children, a special urine collection bag is adhered to the skin surrounding the urethral area. Once the collection is completed, the urine is poured into a collection cup or transferred directly into an evacuated tube with a transfer straw. Urine collected from a diaper is not recommended for laboratory testing since contamination from the diaper material may affect test results.

URINE TESTING

It is possible to discover diseases of many different organs of the body with a urine test. The sample can be taken alone if, for instance, the intention is to find out if you suffer from cystitis. In other cases it will be taken along with other tests (such as stool or blood tests) as part of the investigation process. A urine test is a cheap, simple test that can provide a lot of significant information, for instance:

- Blood in the urine may be a sign of different diseases in the kidneys, the urinary system or the bladder.
- Sugar in the urine may be a sign of diabetes.
- Protein in the urine may be a sign of a kidney disease and can be used to detect the early signs of kidney damage from long-standing diabetes.

NURSING DIAGNOSIS

The following nursing diagnoses are frequently encountered in clients experiencing changes in urinary and bowel habits.

Impaired Urinary Elimination

Impaired Urinary Elimination is the state in which the individual experiences a disturbance in urine elimination. Defining characteristics include dysuria (painful urination), frequency, hesitancy, incontinence, nocturia, retention, and urgency. Altered urinary elimination patterns can result from multiple causes, including anatomic obstruction, sensory motor impairment, and urinary tract infection.

Stress Urinary Incontinence

Stress urinary incontinence is the state in which an individual experiences a loss of urine less than 50 ml occurring with increased abdominal pressure. Major characteristics include reported or observed dribbling with increased abdominal pressure. Minor characteristics may include urinary urgency and urinary frequency (more often than every 2 hours). The client may also be experiencing related factors such as degenerative changes in pelvic muscles and structural supports associated with increased age, high intra-abdominal pressure (e.g., obesity, gravid uterus), incompetent bladder outlet, overdistension between voidings, or weak pelvic muscles and structural supports.

Reflex Urinary Incontinence

The state in which an individual experiences an involuntary loss of urine, occurring at somewhat predictable intervals when a specific bladder volume is reached, is known as Reflex Urinary Incontinence. Major characteristics include no awareness of bladder filling, no urge to void or feelings of bladder fullness, and uninhibited bladder contraction or spasm at regular intervals. Related factors include a neurologic impairment (e.g., spinal cord lesion that interferes with conduction of cerebral messages above the level of the reflex arc).

Urge Urinary Incontinence

Urge Urinary Incontinence is the state in which an individual experiences involuntary passage of urine occurring soon after a strong sense of urgency to void. Major characteristics include urinary urgency, frequency (voiding more often than every 2 hours), and bladder contracture or spasm. Minor characteristics include nocturia (more than two times per night), voiding small amounts (less than 100 ml) or large amounts (more than 550 ml), and inability to reach the toilet in time. Urge incontinence may be related to decreased bladder capacity (e.g., history of pelvic inflammatory disease, abdominal surgeries, indwelling urinary catheter), irritation of bladder stretch receptors causing spasm (e.g., bladder infection), alcohol, caffeine, increased fluids, increased urine concentration, or overdistension of the bladder.

Functional Urinary Incontinence

The state in which an individual experiences an involuntary, unpredictable passage of urine is called Functional Urinary Incontinence. Major characteristics include urge to void or bladder contractions sufficiently strong to result in loss of urine before reaching an appropriate receptacle. Altered environment, sensory, cognitive, or mobility deficits may contribute to functional incontinence.

Total Urinary Incontinence

Total Urinary Incontinence is the state in which an individual experiences a continuous and unpredictable loss of urine. Major characteristics include constant flow of urine occurring at unpredictable times without distension, uninhibited bladder contractions or spasms, unsuccessful incontinence refractory treatments, and nocturia. Related factors include neuropathy that prevents transmission of the reflex that indicates bladder fullness, neurologic dysfunction causing triggering of micturition at unpredictable times, independent contraction of the detrusor reflex owing to surgery, trauma, or disease that affects spinal cord nerves, or anatomy (fistula).

Urinary Retention

The state in which the individual experiences incomplete emptying of the bladder is known as Urinary Retention. Major characteristics for urinary retention include bladder distension and small, frequent voiding or absence of urine output. Minor characteristics include sensation of bladder fullness, dribbling, residual urine, dysuria, and overflow incontinence. High urethral pressure caused by weak detrusor, inhibition of reflex arc, strong sphincter, and blockage are related factors for urinary retention.

BOWEL ELIMINATION

Bowel elimination is a fundamental bodily function that most people carry out in private and are often embarrassed to discuss publicly. Nurses will encounter patients with bowel elimination issues in all areas of care. Knowledge and understanding of both normal function and the problems that can occur with that process will enable nurses to support and care for patients with bowel elimination problems. Here we will discuss the normal anatomy and physiology of elimination, problems, such as faecal incontinence, diarrhoea and constipation, and the nurse's role in their management.

PHYSIOLOGY OF BOWEL ELIMINATION

Five main functions of the bowel are:

- Storage - unabsorbed food residue
- Absorption - Minerals, water, fats

- Secretion - Mucus secreted by the colon to help lubricate the faeces
- Synthesis - Synthesises some vitamins
- Elimination - Propulsion of faecal matter and absorption of fluid

FACTORS AFFECTING BOWEL ELIMINATION

- Poor diet
- Lack of fluid
- Mobility
- Medications
- Surgery

COLLECTION OF SPECIMEN OF FAECES

- Medical aseptic technique is imperative
- Wear disposable gloves
- Wash hands before and after glove use
- Do not contaminate outside of container with stool
- Obtain stool and package, label, and transport according to agency policy

Patient Guidelines

- Void first so urine is not in stool sample
- Defecate into the container rather than toilet bowl
- Do not place toilet tissue in bedpan or specimen container
- Notify nurse when specimen is available
- Get to lab quickly (30 min) if anything viable in sample i.e. parasites, C-diff. etc

FACILITATING BOWEL ELIMINATION

A disposable device for private collection and testing of stool samples of human fecal discharge for the presence of abnormalities such as occult, or hidden blood, which may be a sign of malfunctioning of the intestinal tract of a patient. The device is self-contained and disposable after the test, which can be read by the patient himself. A flexible sample receiving member includes a portion adapted to gravitationally receive an intestinal stool discharge whereby a stool specimen may be deposited in the device and retained in a longitudinally elongated shape during sampling of the stool. After deposition of surface samples of the stool on the surface of the test medium, the stool may be allowed to pass down into the toilet leaving said samples in the device for further test processing. In one such test a reagent can be dispersed longitudinally on the sample, the test "read" by the reaction, if any, of the reagent, the results noted, after which the entire device and stool samples are disposed of without requiring any direct handling or transportation to a laboratory, or the like.

ASSESSMENT

Bowel elimination is infrequent or irregular. Patients describe feeling bloated. The abdomen tympanic and distended and bowel sounds may be hypoactive. The patient experiences rectal fullness, pressure, and pain when he attempts to eradicate the stool. Rectal bleeding may occur as the tissue stretches and tears when the patient tries to pass the hard, dry stool. A comprehensive evaluation of bowel elimination involves collecting data about the patients usual patterns, including frequency of elimination, effort needed to expel stool and what elimination aids.

Equipments

Bedside commode: For an individual who is able to get out of bed but not able to walk to bathroom.

Bedpans: A bedpan is used when an individual is unable to get out of bed at all.

Urinal: An individual uses urinal when he is unable to get out of bed.

PROCEDURES AND SPECIAL CONSIDERATIONS

Expulsion of feces from the rectum and anus

- Faeces enters the rectum
- Stimulates a signal that initiates peristaltic waves in the descending and sigmoid colon and the rectum
- Peristaltic waves force faeces into the anus
- As the peristaltic waves approach the anus, the internal sphincter is inhibited from closing (opened involuntarily)
- Individual senses need to defecate and finds a toilet
- The individual relaxes the external anal sphincter (opened voluntarily)
- Defecation occurs

Enemas: An enema (enemas) is the procedure of introducing liquids into the rectum and colon via the anus. Enemas can be carried out for medical reasons (as a treatment for constipation) as a remedy for encopresis, as part of alternative health therapies, and also for erotic intentions, particularly as part of BDSM activities.

Suppository: A suppository is a drug delivery system that is inserted either into the rectum (rectal suppository), vagina (vaginal suppository) or urethra (urethral suppository) where it dissolves.

Sitz Bath: A Sitz bath (also called a hip bath) is a type of bath in which only the hips and buttocks are soaked in water or saline solution. A Sitz bath is used for patients who have had surgery in the area of the rectum, or to ease the pain of haemorrhoids, uterine cramps, prostate infections, painful ovaries, and/or testicles. It is also used to ease discomfort from infections of the bladder, prostate, or vagina. Inflammatory bowel diseases are also treated with Sitz baths.

Bowel Wash: Bowel wash is performed to keep the body of patients free from bacteria and hazards occurring there from.

Care of Ostomies: The surgery to create the new opening in the abdomen is called ostomy. An ostomy connects either the small or the large intestine to the surface of the body. The opening is called a stoma.

MOBILITY AND IMMOBILITY

Mobility refers to the ability to engage in activity and free movement which includes walking, running, sitting, standing, lifting, pushing, pulling, and performing activities of daily living (ADLs). Mobility is often considered an indicator of health status because it influences the correct functioning of many body systems, especially the respiratory, gastrointestinal, and urinary systems. Mobility enhances muscle tone, increases energy levels, and is associated with psychological benefits such as independence and freedom.

Mobility is regulated by the coordinated effort of the musculoskeletal and neurological systems. The major functions of the musculoskeletal system are to maintain body alignment and to facilitate mobility. The musculoskeletal system consists of a framework of bones, muscles, joints, tendons, ligaments, bursae, and cartilage. The Musculoskeletal System The musculoskeletal system (comprised of bones, cartilage, joints, tendons, ligaments, bursa, and muscles) serves several functions. Bone is the foundation of the musculoskeletal system. Mobility and weight-bearing capacity are directly related to the bone's size and shape. Joints work with muscles to provide motion and flexibility. Skeletal muscles overlying the joint exert opposing forces and, therefore, cause movement.

Posture is maintained primarily by the muscles in the back, neck, trunk, and lower extremities. Nervous System Muscle contraction is controlled by the central nervous system (CNS) and is influenced by the transport of nutrients and oxygen and by the removal of waste products. An intact CNS is essential for coordinated movement to occur. Nerve impulses stimulate the muscles to contract.

The myoneuronal junction is the point at which nerve endings come into contact with muscle cells. The afferent pathway conveys information from sensory receptors to the CNS; these neurons conduct impulses throughout the body. The CNS processes the sensory input and determines a response. The efferent pathway transmits the desired response to skeletal muscles via the somatic nervous system. If the nerve impulses are interrupted, the muscle is paralyzed and cannot contract.

PRINCIPLES OF BODY MECHANICS

Maintain a Stable Centre of Gravity.

- Patients should keep centre of gravity low.
- Patients should keep their back straight.
- Patients should bend at the knees and hips.

Maintain a Wide Base of Support. This will provide the patients with maximum stability while lifting.

- Patients should keep their feet apart.
- Patients should place one foot slightly ahead of the other.
- Patients should flex their knees to absorb jolts.
- Patients should turn with their feet.

Maintain the Line of Gravity. The line should pass vertically through the base of support.

- Patients should keep their back straight.
- Patients should keep the object being lifted close to their body.

Maintain Proper Body Alignment.

- Patients should tuck in their buttocks.
- Patients should pull in their abdomen in and up.
- Patients should keep their back flat.
- Patients should keep their head up.
- Patients should keep their chin in.

- Patients should keep their weight forward and supported on the outside of their feet.

HAZARDS ASSOCIATED WITH IMMOBILITY

Hazards associated with patient immobility have been well documented and are associated with complications involving different organ systems:

- Central nervous: distortion of balance and coordination
- Cardiovascular: reduction of stroke volume and cardiac output, deep vein thrombosis, hypotension
- Gastrointestinal: constipation, glucose intolerance
- Genitourinary: kidney stones, urinary tract infections, reduction of diuresis
- Musculoskeletal: muscle wasting, osteoporosis, pressure lesions
- Respiratory: atelectasis, pneumonia, alveolar derecruitment and extavascular lung volume

REASONS FOR BODY ALIGNMENT AND MOBILITY

The following are reasons for body alignment and mobility.

- To promote comfort and relaxation.
- To restore body function.
- Changing positions improves gastrointestinal function.
- It also improves respiratory function.
- Changing positions allows for greater lung expansion.
- It relieves pressure on the diaphragm.
- To prevent deformities.
- To relieve pressure and prevent strain (which lead to the formation of decubiti).
- To stimulate circulation.
- To give treatments (that is), range of motion exercises).

NURSING INTERVENTION

- Maintain good patient body alignment. Think of the patient in bed as though he were standing.
- Maintain the patient's safety.
- Reassure the patient to promote comfort and cooperation.

- Correctly handle the patient's body to prevent pain or injury.
- Keep in mind proper body mechanics for the practical nurse.
- Obtain assistance, if required, to move heavy or helpless patients.
- Follow specific physician's orders. A physician's order, such as one of the following, is required for the patient to be out of bed.

METHODS AND SPECIAL CONSIDERATIONS

Patients who must lie on their backs much of the time should be kept as comfortable as possible to prevent body deformities. The paraplegic and quadriplegic may not be able to tell the nurse if their position is uncomfortable. Nurses must be especially attentive in this case to prevent possible problems from malalignment.

Pillows can be used to support the patient's head, neck, arms, and hands and a footboard used to support the feet.

- Proper alignment gives respiratory and digestive organs room to function typically.
- The footboard is slanted to support the feet at right angles to the leg (a normal angle) and prevent foot drop.

If the patient's trunk must lie flatter than the neck and head:

- The patient should have only one pillow to support the head and neck.
- The patient may have a pillow placed under the legs to prevent pressure on the heels.

Special Considerations

- Collect equipment.
- Pillows.
- Positioning aids as indicated.
- Nurse should wash her hands correctly.
- She should approach and identify the patient (by checking the identification band) and explain the procedure (using simple terms and pointing out the benefits).
- Provide privacy throughout the procedure.
- Position the bed.

- Place the bed in a flat or level position at working height, unless contraindicated.
- Lower the side rails on the proximal side (as necessary).
- Move the patient from a lateral (side) position to a supine position.
- For the patient on his side, remove supportive pillows.
- Fold top bedding back to the hips, being careful toavoid any undue exposure of the patient's body.
- With one hand on the patient's shoulder and one on the hip, roll his body in one piece (like a log) over onto his back.
- Align the patient's body in good position.
- Head, neck, and spine are in a straight line.
- Arms are at the patient's sides (parallel to the body) with hands prone.
- Legs are parallel to his body.
- Hips, knees, and feet should be in good alignment.
- Support the body parts in good alignment for comfort.
- Place a pillow under the head and shoulders to prevent strain on neck muscles and hyperextension and flexion of the neck.
- Put a footboard at the foot of the bed and place the feet flat against it (at right angles to the legs) to prevent plantar flexion ("foot drop").
- Arrange a sandbag along the outer portion of the right foot to keep the foot upright.
- Make a trochanter roll and arrange it along the right hip and thigh to keep the hip joint from rotating outward.
- Place a pillow under each forearm so the arm is at least six inches from the body.
- Provide for the patient's comfort and safety.
- Replace the bedding neatly and raise the side rails, if used.
- Place the call light within reach.
- Position the bedside stand or overbed table so that the patient will be within easy reach of drinking water and personal items.
- Leave the bed in the low position.
- Report significant nursing observations to the charge nurse.

Rehabilitation Aspects

- Decrease in self-notion and increase in sense of powerlessness due to inability to move purposefully and dependence on someone for assistance with simple self-care activities.
- Body image distortions (depends on diagnosis).
- Decrease in sensory stimulation due to lack of activity, and altered sleep-wake pattern.
- Increased risk of depression, which may cause the patient to become apathetic, possibly because of decreased sensory stimulation; or the patient may exhibit altered thought processes.
- Decreased social interaction.

RANGE OF MOTION EXERCISES

- Passive. These exercises are carried out by the nurse, without assistance from the patient. Passive exercises will not preserve muscle mass or bone mineralization because there is no voluntary contraction, lengthening of muscle, or tension on bones.
- Active Assistive. These exercises are performed by the patient with assistance from the nurse. Active assistive exercises encourage normal muscle function while the nurse supports the distal joint.
- Active. Active exercises are performed by the patient, without assistance, to increase muscle strength.
- Resistive. These are active exercises performed by the patient by pulling or pushing against an opposing force.
- Isometric. These exercises are performed by the patient by contracting and relaxing muscles while keeping the part in a fixed position. Isometric exercises are done to maintain muscle strength when a joint is immobilized. Full patient cooperation is needed.
- Flexion. The state of being bent. The cervical spine is flexed when the chin is moved toward the chest.
- Extension. The state of being in a straight line. The cervical spine is extended when the head is held straight.
- Hyperextension. The state of exaggerated extension. The cervical spine is hyperextended when the individual looks overhead, toward the ceiling.

- Abduction. Lateral movement of a body part away from the midline of the body. The arm is abducted when it is held away from the body.
- Adduction. Lateral movement of a body part toward the midline of the body. The arm is adducted when it is moved from an outstretched position toward the body.
- Rotation. Turning of a body part around an axis. The head is rotated when moved from side to side to indicate "no."
- Circumduction. Rotating an extremity in a complete circle. Circumduction is a combination of abduction, adduction, extension, and flexion.
- Supination. The palm or sole is rotated in an upward position
- Pronation. The palm or sole is rotated in a downward position.

Maintaining Body Alignment: Positions

Moving

In moving the patient nurses should keep in mind that he should not be too far from his bed as in case of his feeling discomfort he can't be bring back to his bed easily.

Lifting

- Use the stronger leg muscles for lifting.
- Bend at the knees and hips; keep your back straight.
- Lift straight upward, in one smooth motion.

Reaching

- Stand directly in front of and close to the object.
- Avoid twisting or stretching.
- Use a stool or ladder for high objects.
- Maintain a good balance and a firm base of support.
- Before moving the object, be sure that it is not too large or too heavy.

Pivoting

- Place one foot slightly ahead of the other.
- Turn both feet at the same time, pivoting on the heel of one foot and the toe of the other.
- Maintain a good centre of gravity while holding or carrying the object.

Avoid Stooping

- Squat (bending at the hips and knees).
- Avoid stooping (bending at the waist).
- Use your leg muscles to return to an upright position.

Transferring

While transferring the patient nurses should make sure that they make patient comfort and he should not be moved unnecessarily as he may feel pain or discomfort.

Walking

While making the patient walk nurses should make sure that some one should always be there to hold the patient as the patient is quite likely to fell down and they should also ensure all other safety measures.

Restraints

- Restraints are anything that restricts a patient's or resident's free movement. The most common are:
- Soft bands used to secure a patient's or resident's wrists or ankles
- Roll belt - secures the midsection

Other restraints include:

- Mittens to secure hands
- Vest restraints, which help immobilize a patient's or resident's upper body
- Swedish belt - secures patient/resident in wheelchair
- Geri chair - reclining chair with a locking tray in front
- Leather bands - have key locks
- Chemical restraints (medications) - used to control behaviour or restrict patient/resident's freedom of movement.

OXYGENATION

Oxygenation refers to the amount of oxygen in a medium. In blood it may be taken to be synonymous with saturation, which describes the degree to which the oxygen-carrying capacity of haemoglobin is utilised, typically 98-100%.

Oxygenation also refers to the process of adding oxygen to a medium such as water or body tissue. Claims have been made that oxygenation of human tissue prevent diseases, including cancer, nevertheless some regard these claims as unverifiable. Oxygenation of various fluorocarbon liquids has been used successfully in liquid breathing systems, allowing air-breathing animals, including humans, to breathe liquids for short periods of time.

PHYSIOLOGY

The delivery of oxygen to the body's cells is a process that depends upon the interplay of the pulmonary, haematological, and cardiovascular systems. Specifically, the processes involved include ventilation, alveolar gas exchange, oxygen transport and delivery, and cellular respiration.

Ventilation

The first step in the process of oxygenation is ventilation, which is the movement of air into and out of the lungs for the purpose of delivering fresh air into the lung's alveoli. Ventilation is regulated by respiratory control centres in the pons and medulla oblongata, which are located in the brain stem. The rate and depth of ventilation are constantly adjusted in response to changes in the concentrations of hydrogen ion (pH) and carbon dioxide (CO2) in the body's fluids. For instance, an increase in carbon dioxide in the blood or a decrease in pH in the body's fluids will stimulate faster and deeper ventilation. A decrease in blood oxygen concentration (hypoxemia) will also stimulate ventilation, but to a lesser degree. Inhalation of air is initiated when the diaphragm contracts, pulling it downward and thus increasing the size of the intrathoracic space. This space is also increased by contraction of the external intercostal muscles, which elevate and separate the ribs and move the sternum forward.

The effect of increasing the space inside the thorax is to decrease the intrathoracic pressure, so that air will be drawn in from the atmosphere. Stretch receptors in the lung tissue send signals back to the brain to cause cessation of inhalation, preventing overdistension of the lungs. Exhalation occurs when the respiratory muscles relax, thus reducing the size of the intrathoracic space, increasing the intrathoracic pressure, and forcing air to exit the lungs. Under normal conditions, exhalation is a passive process. When the movement of air is impeded, additional muscles may be used to increase the ventilatory ability. These accessory muscles of ventilation include the sternocleidomastoid muscle, the abdominal muscles, and the internal intercostal muscles. In some disease states, exhalation is impaired, requiring that the individual actively force air out of the lungs rather than passively exhaling.

Forced expiration is aided by the intercostal muscles and the abdominal recti. When additional muscular force is required for breathing, the work of breathing is said to be increased. Several mechanisms exist to keep the airways clear of micro-organisms and debris.

As air is inhaled through the nose, the larger particles are filtered out through hairs lining the nasal passages. The mucous membranes of the nasopharynx and sinuses warm and humidify the inspired air, and the film of mucus lining these membranes traps smaller particles. Closure of the glottis protects the airway from aspiration of food and fluids during swallowing.

In the trachea and larger bronchi, tiny hairlike cilia continually produce wavelike movements to propel mucus and particles upward, where they can be coughed out. If any invaders manage to reach the alveoli, specialized alveolar macrophages will engulf and destroy the offending organism. Disease processes can interfere with any of these protective mechanisms, increasing the individual's vulnerability to infection and injury.

Alveolar Gas Exchange

Once fresh air reaches the lung's alveoli, the next step in the process of oxygenation begins. The exchange of oxygen from the alveolar space into the pulmonary capillary blood is referred to as oxygen uptake; it may also be called external respiration. Oxygen diffuses across the alveolar membrane in response to a concentration gradient; that is, it moves from an area of higher concentration (the alveoli) to an area of lower concentration (the pulmonary capillary blood), seeking equilibrium. At the same time, carbon dioxide diffuses from the blood to the alveolar space, also in response to a concentration gradient.

FACTORS AFFECTING OXYGENATION

Adequate oxygenation is influenced by many factors, including age, environmental and lifestyle factors, and disease processes.

Age

Oxygenation status can be influenced by age. Older adults may exhibit a barrel chest and require increased effort to expand the lungs. Loss of alveolar gas exchange is accompanied by a decrease in the partial pressure of oxygen. Older adults are also more susceptible to respiratory infection because of decreased activity in the cilia, which normally are an effective defence mechanism.

Environmental and Lifestyle Factors

Environmental and lifestyle factors can significantly affect a client's oxygenation status. Clients who are exposed to dust, animal dander, asbestos, or toxic chemicals in the home or workplace are at increased risk for alterations in oxygenation. Individuals who experience significant physical or emotional stress or who are obese or underweight are also subject to changes in oxygenation status. Smokers and those exposed to second-hand smoke should be questioned as to the type and amount of tobacco and number of years of exposure.

Disease Processes

Oxygenation alterations can often be traced to disease states related to alterations in ventilation, alveolar gas exchange, oxygen uptake, or circulation. There are many disease states that may affect oxygenation, including obstructive pulmonary disease, restrictive pulmonary disease, diffusion defects, ventilation-perfusion mismatching, atherosclerosis, heart failure, anaemia, and alterations in oxygen uptake.

Obstructive Pulmonary Disease: Alterations in ventilation may be related to obstructive or restrictive pulmonary disease. Obstructive pulmonary disease occurs when the airways become partially or completely blocked, diminishing airflow, or the lungs lose some of their elastic recoil, trapping stale air, which should be exhaled. In both cases, the end result is impaired exhalation, air trapping, and difficulty bringing fresh air into the alveoli. The most common obstructive pulmonary diseases are asthma, emphysema, and chronic bronchitis, collectively known as chronic obstructive pulmonary disease (COPD).

Restrictive Pulmonary Disease: Restrictive pulmonary disease represents pathologies that impair the ability of the chest wall and/or lungs to expand during the inspiratory phase of ventilation. This impairment increases the work of breathing and also reduces airflow to the alveoli. A wide variety of disorders cause restrictive lung disease, including pneumonia and pulmonary fibrosis (scarring). Traumatic injury to the thorax or a break in the pleural membrane that surrounds the lungs may also produce restrictive pulmonary dysfunction. The stability of the chest depends upon the rib cage; multiple rib fractures may produce a type of paradoxical chest wall movement called "flail chest" that impedes normal airflow.

The dual-layer pleural membrane also has an important structural function; it helps maintain a negative pressure between its two layers that keeps the lungs from collapsing upon themselves. A break in either layer of the membrane or an abnormal collection of fluid between them interferes with this function, permits alveoli to collapse, and increases the work of breathing. Alveolar collapse, known as atelectasis, can be caused by pleural defects as described above, by compression from a mass such as a tumour, or by occlusion of the small airways by secretions, which prevents air movement into the associated alveoli. Failure of a client to breathe deeply after abdominal surgery may result in atelectasis. Regardless of the cause, atelectasis results in restrictive pulmonary dysfunction and reduces the amount of alveolar- capillary surface area engaged in gas exchange.

Diffusion Defects: Another mechanism of oxygenation impairment is a decrease in the efficiency of gas diffusion from the alveolar space into the pulmonary capillary blood, known as a diffusion defect. This may be caused by thickening of the alveolar-capillary basement membrane or by marked increases in the speed of blood flow through the pulmonary capillary beds, which reduce contact time with the alveoli. Diffusion defects by themselves are uncommon but may coexist with obstructive or restrictive pulmonary disease such as emphysema, pulmonary edema, or fibrosis.

Ventilation-Perfusion Mismatching: Gas exchange across the alveolar-capillary membrane is also influenced by ventilation-perfusion (V/Q) mismatching, or the balance between ventilation and perfusion. The amount of fresh air entering the alveoli (alveolar ventilation) and the amount of blood flow to various regions of the pulmonary capillary network (perfusion) are not uniform throughout the lungs. Due to alterations in position and the effect of gravity, certain zones of lung tissue may have better ventilation or perfusion than others at any given time. An important mechanism of compensation in healthy lung tissue is to produce vasoconstriction or bronchoconstriction as needed to better match ventilation to perfusion or vice versa.

Many disease states, however, produce areas of ventilation-perfusion mismatching that cannot be overcome by compensatory responses. When mismatching occurs, some alveolar regions will be well ventilated but poorly perfused (a condition known as deadspace), while others may be well perfused but poorly ventilated (known as shunting). Alterations in circulation may occur in either the pulmonary or the systemic vasculature and may be localized or generalized. Generalized decreases in pulmonary circulation may be caused by right-sided heart failure or by pathologies in the pulmonary vascular system such as pulmonary hypertension and the resultant pulmonary artery sclerosis. Regional decreases in pulmonary circulation may be related to blockage of a pulmonary artery by an embolus or by regional vasoconstriction.

Atherosclerosis: Alterations in systemic circulation may also be generalized or localized. A common cause of altered arterial circulation is atherosclerosis. This disease is characterized by narrowing and eventual occlusion of the lumen (opening of the arteries) by deposits of lipids, fibrin, and calcium on the interior walls of the arteries. The reduction in blood flow with accompanying oxygen deprivation leads to ischemia (deprivation of blood flow) and eventual infarction (necrosis or death) of the affected tissue. Atherosclerosis in the coronary arteries (coronary heart disease) and the arteries of the brain (cerebral vascular disease) causes myocardial infarction and stroke, respectively, two of the leading causes of death in our society.

Heart Failure: Generalized decreases in tissue perfusion may be caused by left-sided heart failure or by loss of circulating blood volume as may occur with shock or haemorrhage. Heart failure is a condition in which the heart is unable to pump enough blood to meet the metabolic needs of the body; typically, this is accompanied by a backup of blood in the venous circuits (pulmonary and systemic veins), leading to the condition known as congestive heart failure. The increased pressure of the blood in the engorged veins causes fluid to leak out of the associated capillary beds, causing edema in the tissue, including the lungs (pulmonary edema).

Congestive heart failure results in poor arterial perfusion to the body's tissues. This reduction in cardiac output (amount of blood pumped by the heart) may be mild, causing only vague symptoms, or may be profound enough to cause death. Causes of congestive heart failure include myocardial infarction, hypertensive heart disease, and valvular disorders, among others. Loss of circulating blood volume (hypovolemia) may result from massive bleeding, loss of fluid through a wound (such as an extensive burn injury), or severe dehydration.

Anaemia: Another factor that influences oxygenation is the amount of haemoglobin in the blood available to bind with oxygen. A deficiency of haemoglobin (anaemia) may decrease the oxygen-carrying capacity of the blood. A person who is anaemic may have normal SaO2 levels but still continue to experience inadequate tissue oxygenation at the cellular level. Certain poisoning syndromes, most notably carbon monoxide poisoning, mimic anaemia in that they reduce oxygenation by competing with oxygen for binding sites on the haemoglobin molecule.

ALTERATIONS IN OXYGEN UPTAKE

A final factor to consider in the process of oxygenation involves the uptake of oxygen by the body's cells. Certain conditions may impair the cells' ability to take up and utilize oxygen, particularly when the mitochondria are damaged. Cyanide poisoning and severe sepsis impair mitochondrial functioning, rendering the oxygen in arterial blood useless to the cells.

NURSING INTERVENTIONS IN OXYGENATION

- Evaluate respirations: note quality, rate, pattern, depth, and breathing effort. Both rapid, shallow breathing patterns and hypoventilation affect gas exchange. Shallow, "sighless" breathing patterns postsurgery (as a result of effect of anaesthesia, pain, and immobility) reduce lung volume and decrease ventilation.
- Evaluate lung sounds, noting areas of decreased ventilation and the presence of adventitious sounds.
- Evaluate for signs and symptoms of hypoxemia: tachycardia, restlessness, diaphoresis, headache, lethargy, and confusion.
- Evaluate for signs and symptoms of atelectasis: diminished chest excursion, limited diaphragm excursion, bronchial or tubular breath sounds, rales, tracheal shift to affected side. Collapse of alveoli increases physiological shunting.
- Evaluate for signs or symptoms of pulmonary infarction: cough, haemoptysis, pleuritic pain, consolidation, pleural effusion, bronchial breathing, pleural friction rub, and fever.
- Monitor vital signs. With initial hypoxia and hypercapnia, blood pressure (BP), heart rate, and respiratory rate all rise. As the hypoxia and/or hypercapnia becomes more severe, BP may drop, heart rate tends to continue to be rapid with arrhythmias, and respiratory failure may ensue with the patient unable to maintain the rapid respiratory rate.
- Evaluate for changes in orientation and behaviour. Restlessness is an early sign of hypoxia. Chronic hypoxemia may result in cognitive changes such as memory changes.
- Monitor ABGs and note changes. Increasing $PaCO_2$ and decreasing PaO_2 are signs of respiratory failure. As the patient begins to fail, the respiratory rate will decrease and $PaCO_2$ will begin to rise. Some patients, such as those with COPD,

have a significant decrease in pulmonary reserves, and any physiological stress may result in acute respiratory failure.

- Use pulse oximetry to monitor oxygen saturation and pulse rate. Pulse oximetry is a useful tool to detect changes in oxygenation. Oxygen saturation should be maintained at 90% or greater. This tool can be especially helpful in the outpatient or rehabilitation setting where patients at risk for desaturation from chronic pulmonary diseases can monitor the effects of exercise or activity on their oxygen saturation levels. Home oxygen therapy can then be prescribed as indicated. Patients should be assessed for the need for oxygen both at rest and with activity. A higher litre flow of oxygen is generally needed for activity versus rest (e.g., 2 L at rest, and 4 L with activity). Medicare rules for reimbursement for home oxygen require a $PaCO_2$ less than 58 and/or oxygen saturation of 88% or less on room air. Oxygen delivery is then titrated to maintain an oxygen saturation of 90% or greater.
- Evaluate skin colour for development of cyanosis. For cyanosis to be present, 5 g of haemoglobin must desaturate.
- Monitor chest x-ray reports. Chest x-rays may guide the etiological components of the impaired gas exchange. Keep in mind that radiographic studies of lung water lag behind clinical presentation by 24 hours.
- Monitor effects of position changes on oxygenation (SaO_2, ABGs, SVO_2, and end-tidal CO_2). Putting the most congested lung areas in the dependent position (where perfusion is greatest) potentiates ventilation and perfusion imbalances.
- Evaluate patient's ability to cough effectively to clear secretions. Note quantity, colour, and consistency of sputum. Retained secretions impair gas exchange.

MAINTENANCE OF PATIENT AIRWAY

In the initial evaluation and management of any critically ill patient the ABC's (Airway, Breathing and Circulation) are the first priority. The ability to establish and maintain an open airway in a patient, and the ability to ensure adequate ventilation and oxygenation of the patient, are hence essential skills for nurses. For the intentions of this module "fundamental airway management" will refer to those fundamental interventions that maintain an open airway and assist ventilation but do not include endotracheal intubation.

It is of course significant that physicians be able to recognize when a patient is not adequately ventilating their chest. The reasons for inadequate chest ventilation include inadequate respiratory effort, airway obstruction or a combination of these two. If the patient is not breathing at all (apneic) then the nurses must immediately perform a simple manoeuvre such as a chin lift to open the airway and commence ventilation of the chest with a bag-mask device.

If the patient is making respiratory effort but is not adequately ventilating their chest because of airway obstruction the nurses must determine the cause and take immediate measures to alleviate the obstruction. In an unconscious patient often the cause of the obstruction will be prolapse of the tongue into the posterior pharynx due to loss of tone in the submandibular muscles. This problem can be quickly corrected using a simple manoeuvre such as a head tilt-chin lift or jaw thrust and this may be all that is required to open the airway and allow adequate chest ventilation. If the physician encounters noisy or "gurgling" respirations at this point the upper airway should be suctioned for vomitus and excess secretions.

Simple Airway Manoeuvres

Head Tilt-Chin Lift: This manoeuvre should only be used if the physician is confident there is no risk of injury to the c-spine. Standing on the patient's right hand side, the physician's left hand is used to apply pressure to the forehead to extend the neck. The volar surfaces of the tips of the index and middle finger are used to elevate the mandible which will lift the tongue from the posterior pharynx.

Jaw Thrust: Where there is risk of c-spine injury, such as a patient who is unconscious as a result of a head injury, the airway should be opened using a manoeuvre that does not require neck movement. The jaw thrust is performed by having the physician stand at the head of the patient looking down at the patient. The middle finger of the right hand is placed at the angle of the patient's jaw on the right. The middle finger of the left hand is similarly placed at the angle of the jaw on the left. An upward pressure is applied to elevate the mandible which will lift the tongue from the posterior pharynx.

Airway Adjuncts: Once an open airway has been established the nurse may choose to use either an oropharyngeal or nasopharyngeal airway to make it easier to maintain an open airway. Both of these devices prevent the tongue from occluding the airway and thereby provide an open conduit for air to pass. It is significant to note that these two airway devices, unlike a cuffed endotracheal, tube will not protect the trachea from aspiration of secretions or stomach contents. If a patient is unable to protect their own airway they should have an endotracheal tube inserted as soon as possible by someone who is has specific training and expertise in that skill.

Oropharyngeal airway: The oropharyngeal airway is essentially a curved hollow tube that is used to create an open conduit through the mouth and posterior pharynx. A rough guide for choosing the correct size is to hold the airway beside the patient's mandible, orienting it with the flange at the patient's mouth and the tip at the angle of jaw. The tip should just reach the angle of the jaw.

While inserting the airway you want to avoid pushing the tongue into the posterior pharynx. This can be accomplished by starting with the curve of the airway inverted, and then rotate the airway as the tip reaches the posterior pharynx. Alternatively a tongue depressor can be used to move the tongue out of the way as the airway is passed. Whichever technique is chosen the physician must be certain that the airway is indeed in the right position. If there are problems ventilating the patient after insertion of the airway then it should be removed and reinserted.

Nasopharyngeal airway: The nasopharyngeal airway is a soft rubber or plastic hollow tube that is passed through the nose into the posterior pharynx. The tubes come in sizes based on the internal diameter(i.d.) of the tube. The larger the internal diameter the longer the tube. An 8.0 - 9.0 i.d. is used for a large adult, a 7.0 - 8.0 i.d. for a medium adult and a 6.0 - 7.0 i.d. for a small adult. These tubes can be used when the use of an oropharyngeal airway is difficult, such as when a patient is clenching their jaw. As well, the nasopharyngeal airway is generally better tolerated than the oropharyngeal airway in a semiconscious patient. To insert, the nasopharyngeal airway is lubricated with water soluble lubricant or anaesthetic jelly along the floor of the nostril into posterior pharynx behind the tongue.

SPECIAL CONSIDERATIONS

Maintain oxygen administration device as ordered, attempting to maintain oxygen saturation at 90% or greater. This provides for adequate oxygenation. Avoid high concentration of oxygen in patients with COPD. Hypoxia stimulates the drive to breathe in the chronic CO_2 retainer patient. When applying oxygen, close monitoring is imperative to prevent unsafe increases in the patient's PaO_2, which could result in apnea.

If the patient is allowed to eat, oxygen still must be given to the patient but in a different manner (e.g., changing from mask to a nasal cannula). Eating is an activity and more oxygen will be consumed than when the patient is at rest. Immediately after the meal, the original oxygen delivery system should be returned.

For patients who should be ambulatory, provide extension tubing or portable oxygen apparatus. These promote activity and facilitate more effective ventilation. Position with proper body alignment for optimal respiratory excursion (if tolerated, head of bed at 45 degrees). This promotes lung expansion and improves air exchange.

- Routinely check the patient's position so that he or she does not slide down in bed. This would cause the abdomen to compress the diaphragm, which would cause respiratory embarrassment.
- Position patient to facilitate ventilation/perfusion matching. Use upright, high-Fowler's position whenever possible. High-Fowler's position allows for optimal diaphragm excursion. When patient is positioned on side, the good side should be down (e.g., lung with pulmonary embolus or atelectasis should be up).
- Pace activities and schedule rest periods to prevent fatigue. Even simple activities such as bathing during bed rest can cause fatigue and increase oxygen consumption.
- Change patient's position every 2 hours. This facilitates secretion movement and drainage.
- Suction as required. Suction clears secretions if the patient is unable to effectively clear the airway.
- Encourage deep breathing, using incentive spirometer as indicated. This reduces alveolar collapse.
- For postoperative patients, assist with splinting the chest. Splinting optimizes deep breathing and coughing efforts.
- Encourage or assist with ambulation as indicated. This promotes lung expansion, facilitates secretion clearance, and stimulates deep breathing.
- Provide reassurance and allay anxiety:
- Have an agreed-on method for the patient to call for assistance (e.g., call light, bell).

- Stay with the patient during episodes of respiratory distress.
- Anticipate need for intubation and mechanical ventilation if patient is unable to maintain adequate gas exchange. Early intubation and mechanical ventilation are recommended to prevent full decompensation of the patient. Mechanical ventilation provides supportive care to maintain adequate oxygenation and ventilation to the patient. Treatment also needs to focus on the underlying causal factor leading to respiratory failure.
- Administer medications as prescribed. The type depends on the etiological factors of the problem (e.g., antibiotics for pneumonia, bronchodilators for COPD, anticoagulants/ thrombolytics for pulmonary embolus, analgesics for thoracic pain).

PSYCHOSOCIAL NEEDS

Psychosocial support has been defined as an ongoing process of meeting emotional, social, mental and spiritual needs, all of which are considered essential elements of meaningful and positive human development. Uncertainty escalates anxiety. Explain procedures, telling the client what is expected and what is going to occur. All clients in every health care setting need clear statements of expected behaviour.

The following nursing actions promote the client's psychological safety:

- Respect a client's privacy. Loss of privacy triggers anxiety in most persons. During treatment in any setting, personal probing questions must be asked; procedures often violate physical space and can be offensive; elimination activities often occur in the presence of others. Be sure to protect privacy as much as possible.
- Treat each client as an individual worthy of dignity. This means being sensitive to the feelings of others and recognizing that their feelings may differ from yours and those of other clients.
- Encourage the client to be as independent as possible while providing assistance as required.

Nursing interventions for role change due to deficits in activity and mobility include (1) fostering open family communication, (2) providing opportunities for family role resumption, (3) prioritizing family roles and duties, and (4) modifying family roles and duties.

REFERENCES

Alfaro-LeFevre, R. (1998). Critical thinking in nursing: A practical approach (2nd ed.). Philadelphia: Saunders.

Barnum, B. S., & Kerfoot, K. M. (1995). The nurse as executive (4th ed., pp. 236–248). Gaithersburg, MD: Aspen.

Carpenito, L. J. (1999). Nursing diagnosis: Application to clinical practice (7th ed.). New York: Lippincott.

Jennings, B. M. & Staggers, N. (1999). A provocative look at performance measurement. Nursing Administration Quarterly, 24(1), 17–30.

Joel, L. (1984). Self-regulation protects nursing's growing edge. The American Nurse, 16(2), 4, 22.

Johnson, M., & Maas, M. (Eds.). (1999). Nursing outcomes classification (NOC): Iowa outcome project. St. Louis: Mosby.

Kenney, J. W. (1995). Evaluation. In P. J. Christensen & J. W. Kenney (Eds.), Nursing process: Application of conceptual models (4th ed., pp. 195–207). St. Louis: Mosby.

Murrary, R. B., & Zentner, J. P. (1997). Nursing assessment and health promotion: Strategies through the life span (6th ed., pp. 108–109). Norwalk, CT: Appleton & Lange.

Wakefield, D. S., Helms, C. M., & Helms, L. (1995). The peer review process: The art of judgment. Journal of Healthcare Quality, 17(3), 11–15.

10

Infection Control in Health-Care Setting

Infection control and health care epidemiology is the discipline concerned with preventing the spread of infections within the health-care setting. As such, it is a practical (rather than an academic) sub-discipline of epidemiology. It is an essential (though often underrecognized and undersupported) part of the infrastructure of health care. Infection control and hospital epidemiology are akin to public health practice, practiced within the confines of a particular health-care delivery system rather than directed at society as a whole.

INFECTION CONTROL

Infection control concerns itself both with prevention (hand hygiene/ hand washing, cleaning/disinfection/sterilization, vaccination, surveillance) and with investigation and management of demonstrated or suspected spread of infection within a particular health-care setting (e.g. outbreak investigation). It is on this basis that the common title being adopted within health care is "Infection Prevention & Control".

The nurse plays a critical role in preventing and controlling infectious disease. The beginning nursing student participates significantly in the prevention process from the initial introduction to nursing care.

A significant component in preparing for clinical nursing practice is an understanding of the infection process and prevention techniques. Microbiology and other science courses provide background information about pathogenic organisms. The transfer of these scientific principles to the applied art and science of nursing involves an awareness of the dynamics of the infectious process.

FACTORS

The presence of infectious micro organisms and an individual's weakened health condition are two contributing factors to the infection process. Illness and injury influence the body's ability to resist pathogenic micro organisms. Lowered resistance to micro organisms occurs under conditions of poor nutritional status, open wounds, invasive therapies, or a suppressed immune system. These conditions, associated with illness and injury, become more dangerous when the patient is very old or very young. Within the health care setting the number of infected or colonized persons is quite high. As a result, the health care setting is an environment rich in pathogenic micro organisms.

Antibiotic therapy, the primary medical treatment for infection, also promotes a great danger: the development of drug-resistant strains of micro organisms, such as MRSA or VRE. Many of these organisms colonize in a host without causing an acute infection. Colonization is the presence and multiplication of a micro organism without tissue invasion or damage. A patient with micro organism colonization does not show signs of infection and is not immediately recognized as a reservoir of an infectious agent.

CHAIN OF INFECTION TRANSMISSION

Infectious Agent: A microbial organism with the ability to cause disease. The greater the organism's virulence (ability to grow and multiply), invasiveness (ability to enter tissue) and pathogenicity (ability to cause disease), the greater the possibility that the organism will cause an infection. Infectious agents are bacteria, viruses, fungi, and parasites.

Reservoir: A place within which micro organisms can thrive and reproduce. For instance, micro organisms thrive in human beings, animals, and inanimate objects such as water, table tops, and doorknobs.

Portal of Exit: A place of exit providing a way for a micro organism to leave the reservoir. For instance, the micro organism may leave the reservoir through the nose or mouth when someone sneezes or coughs. Micro organisms, carried away from the body by feces, may also leave the reservoir of an infected bowel.

Mode of Transmission: Method of transfer by which the organism moves or is carried from one place to another. The hands of the health care worker may carry bacteria from one individual to another.

Portal of Entry: An opening allowing the micro organism to enter the host. Portals include body orifices, mucus membranes, or breaks in the skin. Portals also result from tubes placed in body cavities, such as urinary catheters, or from punctures produced by invasive procedures such as intravenous fluid replacement.

Susceptible Host: An individual who cannot resist a micro organism invading the body, multiplying, and resulting in infection. The host is susceptible to the disease, lacking immunity or physical resistance to overcome the invasion by the pathogenic micro organism.

DEFENCES AGAINST INFECTION

Natural defences against infection control is that which has been inherited in contrast to one that has been acquired. If an individual acquires immunity by having the disease in question, as opposed to acquiring it as the result of vaccination, then that individual is said to have natural acquired immunity.

As long ago as the 5th century B.C., Greek physicians noted that people who had recovered from the plague would never get it again-they had acquired immunity. This is because, whenever T cells and B cells are activated, some of the cells become "memory" cells. Then, the next time that an individual encounters that same antigen, the immune system is primed to destroy it quickly.

The degree and duration of immunity depend on the kind of antigen, its amount, and how it enters the body. An immune response is also dictated by heredity; some persons respond strongly to a given antigen, others weakly, and some not at all.

Infants are born with relatively weak immune responses. They have, nevertheless, a natural "passive" immunity; they are protected during the first months of life by means of antibodies they receive from their mothers. The antibody IgG, which travels across the placenta, makes them immune to the same microbes to which their mothers are immune. Children who are nursed also receive IgA from breast milk; it protects the digestive tract.

Passive immunity can also be conveyed by antibody-containing serum obtained from persons who are immune to a specific infectious agent. Immune serum globulin or "gamma globulin" is sometimes given to protect travellers to countries where hepatitis is widespread. Passive immunity normally lasts only a few weeks.

"Active" immunity-mounting an immune response-can be triggered by both infection and vaccination. Vaccines contain micro-organisms that have been altered so they will produce an immune response but will not be able to induce full-blown disease. Some vaccines are made from microbes that have been killed. Others use microbes that have been changed slightly so they can no longer produce infection. They may, for instance, be unable to multiply. Some vaccines are made from a live virus that has been weakened, or attenuated, by growing it for many cycles in animals or cell cultures.

Recent research, benefiting from the biotechnology revolution, has focused on developing vaccines that use only part of the infectious agent. Such subunit vaccines, which are now available for meningitis, pneumonia, and hepatitis B, produce the desired immunity without stirring up separate and potentially harmful immune reactions to the many antigens carried, for instance, on a single bacterium.

HOSPITAL ACQUIRED INFECTION

Nosocomial infections are infections which are a result of treatment in a hospital or a healthcare service unit, but secondary to the patient's original condition (and as such are a category of iatrogenic artefacts). Infections are considered nosocomial if they first appear 48 hours or more after hospital admission or within 30 days after discharge. Nosocomial comes from the Greek word nosokomeion. This type of infection is also known as a hospital-acquired infection (or more generically healthcare-associated infections).

Nosocomial infections are even more alarming in the 21st century. The main reasons are the followings:

- Hospitals house large numbers of people who are sick and whose immune systems are often in a weakened state.
- Increased use of outpatient treatment means that people who are in the hospital are sicker on average.
- Medical staff move from patient to patient, providing a way for pathogens to spread.
- Many medical procedures bypass the body's natural protective barriers.
- Sanitation protocol regarding uniforms, equipment sterilization, washing, and other preventative measures may be either unheeded by hospital staff or too lax to sufficiently isolate patients from infectious agents.
- Patients are often prescribed antibiotics and other anti-microbial drugs to help treat illness; this may increase the selection pressure for the emergence of resistant strains.

Thorough hand washing and/or use of alcohol rubs by all medical personnel before each patient contact is one of the most effective ways to combat nosocomial infections. More careful use of anti-microbial agents, such as antibiotics, is also considered vital.

Micro-organisms are transmitted in hospitals by several routes, and the same micro-organism may be transmitted by more than one route. There are five main routes of transmission: contact, droplet, airborne, common vehicle, and vector-borne.

Contact transmission: The most important and frequent mode of transmission of nosocomial infections, is divided into two subgroups: direct-contact transmission and indirect-contact transmission.

- Direct-contact transmission: It involves a direct body surface-to-body surface contact and physical transfer of micro-organisms between a susceptible host and an infected or colonized person, such as occurs when a person turns a patient, gives a patient a bath, or performs other patient-care activities that require direct personal contact. Direct-contact transmission also can occur between two patients, with one serving as the source of the infectious micro-organisms and the other as a susceptible host.
- Indirect-contact transmission involves contact of a susceptible host with a contaminated intermediate object, usually inanimate, such as contaminated instruments, needles, or dressings, or contaminated gloves that are not changed between patients. Additionally, the improper use of saline flush syringes, vials, and bags have been implicated in disease transmission in the US, even when healthcare workers had access to gloves, disposable needles, intravenous devices, and flushes.

Droplet transmission occurs when droplets are generated from the source person mainly during coughing, sneezing, and talking, and during the performance of certain procedures such as bronchoscopy. Transmission occurs when droplets containing germs from the infected person are propelled a short distance through the air and deposited on the host's body.

- Airborne transmission occurs by dissemination of either airborne droplet nuclei (small-particle residue {5 μm or smaller in size} of evaporated droplets containing micro-organisms that remain suspended in the air for long periods of time) or dust particles containing the infectious agent. Micro-organisms carried in this manner can be dispersed widely by air currents and may become inhaled by a susceptible host within the same room or over a longer distance from the source patient, depending on environmental factors; therefore, special air handling and ventilation are required to prevent airborne transmission. Micro-organisms transmitted by airborne transmission include Legionella, Mycobacterium tuberculosis and the rubeola and varicella viruses.

- Common vehicle transmission applies to micro-organisms transmitted to the host by contaminated items such as food, water, medications, devices, and equipment.

ASEPSIS

Asepsis is the practice to reduce or eradicate contaminants (such as bacteria, viruses, fungi, and parasites) from entering the operative field in surgery or medicine to prevent infection. Ideally, a field is "sterile" - free of all contaminants - a situation that is difficult to attain. However, elimination of infection is the goal of asepsis, not sterility.

Medical asepsis is a clean technique used to reduce and prevent the spread of micro-organisms. Surgical asepsis is a sterile technique that requires nurses to use different precautions than they do for medical asepsis. It includes procedures used to eradicate all micro-organisms, including pathogens and spores, from an object or area. Surgical asepsis procedures are followed when performing an invasive procedure into a body cavity typically free of micro-organisms. Medical aspesis means clean; surgical asepsis means sterile.

A sterile object remains sterile only when touched by another sterile object. Only sterile objects may be placed on a sterile field. A sterile object or field out of the range of vision or an object held below a person's waist is contaminated. The edges of a sterile field or container are considered contaminated. A sterile object or field becomes contaminated by prolonged exposure to air. When a sterile surface comes in contact with a wet contaminated surface, the sterile object or field becomes contaminated by capillary action.

Asepsis means absence of disease producing organisms. The micro-organisms of different types are present everywhere in our environment and in the human body. The intention of medical asepsis is to prevent by all means of cross-infections from one patient to another, including communicable disease infections. The intention of surgical asepsis is to prevent by all means of infections of the wounds of surgical patients, infection of the uterus during and after delivery, and infection that could be introduced by invasive procedures such as catheterisation, injections and infusions.

MEDICAL ASEPSIS

This includes:

- General cleanliness
- Isolation of infected persons.
- Disinfection of all articles that may be contaminated, or used for more than one patient.
- Correct and frequent hand-washing by all those caring for patients.

Hand-washing Technique

- Wet the hands under running water.
- Apply soap thoroughly, and use a brush for the nails if possible.
- Rinse well.
- Dry with a clean towel. It is significant to keep the nails short.

Use of Gowns, Gloves and Masks, in Medical Asepsis

Any patient who is a source of infection needs to be isolated. The type of isolation depends on the method by which the organisms may spread from individual to individual.

Gown: Gown protection is required for persons in close contact with a patient who may spread infection by urine, faeces, vomit, or wound drainage. (e.g.) typhoid fever, dysentery, cholera, gas gangrene.

At the entrance to the patients unit a stand should be provided on which to hang the isolation gown. If the stand is inside the unit, the gown is hung with the contaminated side out.

- If outside the unit, it is hung clean side out.
- To put on the gown, insert your hands into the sleeves of the gown without touching the contaminated side.
- Then fasten the neck-band, which is considered clean. Fasten the belt and then carry out the work in the unit.
- After finishing, untie the belt, wash your hands and untie the neckband.

- Remove the first sleeve, remove the second sleeve by grasping it with the gown-covered hand.
- Place the gown carefully on the hook, then wash your hands again thoroughly.

Gloves: This is required to protect persons coming in close contact with a patient having a communicable disease, which is air-borne. (e.g) diphtheria, sore throat, meningitis, chickenpox, whooping cough etc. In most of these cases a gown is also required.

Clean gloves are commonly adequate in medical asepsis, but when handling a wound after surgery or the vagina during delivery or in the puerperium, sterile gloves are required. After using the gloves, they are removed and placed into a disinfectant solution. The gloved hands may be washed under the running water before taking them off and then placed in the disinfectant solution.

Use of Masks: Clean masks should be kept in a clean area near the hand-washing facilities at the entrance of the isolation unit. Take a mask and tie it on before you enter. When leaving, wash hands, remove the mask holding the strings only, and drop it into a second container for used masks. Masks must be disinfected before being used again. Now disposable masks are available for use and throw.

Isolation Technique

- The degree of isolation will depend on the type of disease.
- The patient should be isolated as long as he/she is a source of infection. The time depends on the particular disease.
- Persons attending the patient should be limited to one or two and no visitors allowed.
- The room should have only essential furniture and be easily cleaned (Damp dusting and floor cleaning).
- Gown, apron and mask should be provided for any one entering the room. Used masks are to be dropped into disinfectant solution.
- Hands should be washed with soap and water after touching the patient. All the articles used by him should be disinfected
- Everything taken out of the room must be disinfected. Dust, excreta and discharges, waste food soiled linen and utensils, must be disposed off with care.

- For terminal disinfection, the patient is given a bath and clean clothes, and taken away from the isolation room. Then the room and everything in it is thoroughly disinfected.

Barrier Nursing

In this type of isolation, the corner of a general medical ward is suitable for patient with infections other than air-borne. (e.g) Typhoid fever, dysentery and diarrhoea. It is best if the room is screened against flies. A gown or apron and hand washing facilities are kept at the bedside. Excreta must be carefully disposed of bedpans and bed linen is disinfected. All other precautions are taken to prevent the spread of the infections.

SURGICAL ASEPSIS

This means keeping objects and areas 'sterile' free from all organisms. Surgical asepsis (Sterile technique) is used in the operating room, delivery room, in doing surgical dressings and many other invasive procedures. The nurse must thoroughly understand the principle of surgical asepsis. She must be reliable in always keeping to these principles. She must know about the use and care of the masks, gloves and gowns, the proper technique of hand washing for surgical procedures and the sterilizing and handling of sterile equipments.

Masks, Gloves and Gowns for Surgical Use

Masks: A facemask is worn when doing any sterile surgical procedures. The intention of the mask in surgical nursing is to prevent any germs from the person's respiratory tract from being breathed up on the wound or sterile articles.

- The mask should cover both nose and mouth of the wearer.
- It is made of two or more layers of material, either in rectangular or nosebag shape, with tapes to tie at the back of head.
- While being worn, the face piece should not be touched.
- If it becomes wet with sweat or by sneezing, it should be changed.
- Do not speak more than necessary during surgery.
- A fresh mask should be worn for each procedure.
- The mask should neither be suspended around the neck nor put into the pocket.
- After use, remove the mask, hold it by the tapes, and place it straight into antiseptic solution.

- At the end of each day, the used masks should be washed, dried, then folded with tapes outside and sterilized ready for use again.
- In some hospitals, disposable masks are worn.

Gloves: Surgical gloves in various sizes are made of special thin rubber so that the surgeon may not lose the sense of touch.

- In clean operations they are worn to protect the patient, but in infected cases they protect the wearer also.
- After use, gloves should be washed in cold water and then with soap and water.
- By filling the glove with water holes can be detected.
- The gloves may be wiped dry or hung on a rack and turned to dry the inside as well.
- To prepare for sterilizing, dust the gloves well both inside and out with glove powder.
- See that the roughened surface is on the outside (for better grip) then pair off the gloves.
- Turn back the cuffs 5 cm and place a small pocket of glove powder just inside the right-hand glove.
- Place the pair of gloves in a glove pocket marked with the correct size. Disposable gloves are now in use.

Gowns: Steam sterilized theatre gowns are worn by the scrubbed-up operating team, to prevent contamination of the sterile field by the contact with clothing or skin. Unsterile but clean gowns are often worn by those persons in the operating room who are not scrubbed up.

- For the surgeon and his assistant particularly, gowns should be made of close- woven material.
- For all those scrubbed up, the gowns must have sleeves, which are long enough to fit under the gloves at the wrists.
- All the gowns fasten at the back.
- An unsterile helper ties the tapes without touching the outside of the sterile gown.
- After use, gowns are soaked in cold water if blood stained, then hung to dry and sent to the laundry, or well washed in hot soapy water and ironed.

- Gowns to be sterilized must be folded and rolled up in such a way that only the inner surface is handled by the scrubbed up persons.
- They are packed in drums or bundles ready for autoclaving.

Method of using sterile gowns and gloves:

- Take hold of the gown at arms length with your scrubbed up hands, unroll, and slip arms into the smaller, asking a helper to the tapes at the back. Both you and the helper must be very careful not to touch the outside of the gown.
- Dust your hands with sterile powder, and put on the gloves. Hold the first glove by the turned back cuff, and slip it on. Next insert the gloved fingers under the cuff of the second glove and slip it on. The cuff of each glove is then unfolded and pulled completely over the sleeve end of the gown. These must be no gap at the wrist, and the nurse must not touch the bare skin nor inside of glove or gown when scrubbed up.
- The first scrubbed up individual may help others by holding the sterile gloves for them to slip in their hands. When scrubbed up, the nurse must remember to touch only sterile things. The instrument table and whole field of operation is draped with large sterile clothes and towels. Helpers who are not scrubbed up may help to bring sterile suppliers to the tables, keeping to the outside and using 'Cheatle forceps'.

Caps, clothing and footwear: In the operating theatre, there must be no risk of introducing dust and dirt, especially any soil that may contain tetanus organisms. Therefore every individual entering must wear clean clothing, and put on clean theatre slippers or canvas shoes.

- These must be removed on leaving the theatre.
- The hair must be completely covered by means of a clean theatre cap.

Surgical hand-scrub: In all surgical work it is significant to keep the hands and nails clean. Nails must be cut or filed very short.

- The surgical hand scrub is necessary for the surgeons and those assisting at an operation, and for sterile procedures.
- It must be realized that hands can never be made sterile except by wearing sterile gloves.

In surgical hand scrub requirements are:

- Running water.
- Antiseptic soap or soap solution.
- Sterile nail brush
- Sterile towel.

Method of surgical hand scrub is:

- Wear a clean cap and then a clean mask.
- Note the time, the procedure should take 10 minutes.
- Wet the hands up to the elbows under the running water.
- Apply soap to make a good lather, and look it into the hands and arms, adding small amounts of water but not enough to remove the lather.
- After 30 seconds, rinse thoroughly.
- Apply more soap and this time uses the brush. Pay special attention to the nails, fingertips and between fingers. Add more water in small amounts frequently but keep the lather, with more soap also. After the nails, fingers and hand, work up the arm, scrubbing gently with circular motions and following at the elbow. Repeat for the other arm.
- Rinse the arms and other hands with forearms held up so that water does not run down from the elbows to the hands.
- Dry on a sterile towel, starting with the hands and moving upwards.

TRANSPORTATION OF INFECTED PATIENTS

Appropriate patient transportation is a significant component of isolation precautions. A private room is significant to prevent direct or indirect contact transmission when the source patient has poor hygienic habits, contaminates the environment, or cannot be expected to assist in maintaining infection control precautions to limit transmission of micro-organisms (i.e., infants, children, and patients with altered mental status).

When possible, a patient with highly transmissible or epidemiologically significant micro-organisms is placed in a private room with hand washing and toilet facilities, to reduce opportunities for transmission of micro-organisms.

When a private room is not available, an infected patient is placed with an appropriate roommate. Patients infected by the same micro-organism commonly can share a room, provided they are not infected with other potentially transmissible micro-organisms and the likelihood of reinfection with the same organism is minimal. Such sharing of rooms, also referred to as cohorting patients, is useful especially during outbreaks or when there is a shortage of private rooms.

Guidelines for construction, equipment, air handling, and ventilation for isolation rooms have been delineated in other publications. A private room with appropriate air handling and ventilation is particularly significant for reducing the risk of transmission of micro-organisms from a source patient to susceptible patients and other persons in hospitals when the micro-organism is spread by airborne transmission.

Limiting the movement and transport of patients infected with virulent or epidemiologically significant micro-organisms and ensuring that such patients leave their rooms only for essential intentions reduces opportunities for transmission of micro-organisms in hospitals. When patient transport is necessary, it is significant that (1) appropriate barriers (e.g., masks, impervious dressings) are worn or used by the patient to reduce the opportunity for transmission of pertinent micro-organisms to other patients, personnel, and visitors and to reduce contamination of the environment; (2) personnel in the patient and of the patient is to be taken are notified of the impending arrival of the patient and of the precautions to be used to reduce the risk of transmission of infectious micro-organisms; and, (3) patients are informed of ways by which they can assist in preventing the transmission of their infectious micro-organisms to others.

BIOMEDICAL WASTE MANAGEMENT

Hospitals are one of the complex institutions which are frequented by people from every walk of life in the society without any distinction between age, sex, race and religion. This is over and above the normal inhabitants of hospital i.e., patients and staff. All of them produce waste which is increasing in its amount and type due to advances in scientific knowledge and is creating its impact. The hospital waste, in addition to the risk for patients and personnel who handle these wastes poses a threat to public health and environment. Keeping in view inappropriate biomedical waste management, the Ministry of Environment and Forests notified the "Biomedical Waste (management and handling) Rules, 1998" in July 1998. In accordance with these Rules (Rule 4), it is the duty of every "occupier" i.e., an individual who has the control over the institution and or its premises, to take all steps to ensure that waste generated is handled without any adverse effect to human health and environment. The hospitals, nursing homes, clinic, dispensary, animal house, pathological lab etc., are hence needed to set in place the biological waste treatment facilities. It is nevertheless not incumbent that every institution has to have its own waste treatment facility. The rules also envisage that common facility or any other facilities can be used for waste treatment. However it is incumbent on the occupier to ensure that the waste is treated within a period of 48 hours.

TYPES OF HOSPITAL WASTE

Large quantities of hospital waste are produced every day from a wide range of sources. Clinical waste can be classified according to a number of categories, depending on its source. Clinical waste is defined by the Controlled Waste Regulations (1992) as any waste that consists wholly or partly of:

- Blood or other bodily fluids
- Drugs or other pharmaceutical products
- Excretions
- Human or animal tissue
- Swabs or dressings
- Syringes, needles or other sharp instruments which, unless made safe, may be hazardous to anybody who comes in contact with it.

Examples of clinical waste include:

- Any item which is or may be soiled by blood or body fluids
- Colostomy and urine bags
- Empty IV bags and administration sets
- Human tissue
- Incontinence bags
- Pharmaceutical waste
- Vomit bowls and sputum pots
- Waste arising from treatments using cytotoxic drugs.

The principal sources of clinical waste are:

- Blood transfusion centres

- Dental surgeries
- GPs' surgeries
- Health centres
- Hospitals
- Research establishments
- Public health laboratories
- Veterinary surgeries.

Unless clinical waste is correctly segregated, handled, transported and disposed of it can present risks to the health and safety of people at work, members of the public, and the environment.

HAZARDS ASSOCIATED WITH HOSPITAL WASTE

There are many examples and ample evidences that indiscriminate management of Bio-Medical Waste could cause serious hazards to health and environment as follows

- There are many harmful agents in the Biomedical waste. The most important are Biological agents, which pollute water and food and cause alimentary infections like cholera, typhoid, dysentery, infective hepatitis, polio, ascariasis and hook worm diseases etc.
- Wastes breed vermin and pests. Examples are: a. Mosquitoes that transmit insect borne diseases like malaria and filaria. b. Common house flies which transmit infections mechanically. c. Many other insects and worms that cause nuisance e.g. cockroaches, ants. d. Rats thriving on refuse.
- Dust may harbour Tubercle Bacilli and other germs, which cause diseases if inhaled.
- Soil polluted by night soil may be rich in Tetanus spores.
- Nosocomiol infections and AIDS, Hepatitis B&C etc.
- Aesthetic: Sullage water, refuse and night soil, all create intolerable nuisance of sight and smell.

BIOMEDICAL WASTE MANAGEMENT PROCESS

Handling, segregation, mutilation, disinfection, storage, transportation and final disposal are vital steps for safe and scientific management of biomedial waste in any establishment. The key to minimisation and effective management of biomedical waste is segregation (separation) and identification of the waste. The most appropriate way of identifying the categories of biomedical waste is by sorting the waste into colour coded plastic bags or containers. Biomedical waste incineration, autoclave, hydroclave or microwave.

COST OF BIOMEDICAL WASTE MANAGEMENT

The cost of construction, operation and maintenance of system for managing biomedical waste represents a significant part of overall budget of a hospital if the BMW handling rules 1998 have to be implemented in their true spirit. Govt. of India in its pilot project for hospital waste management in Govt. hospitals has estimated Rs.85 lakh as capital cost in 1000 bedded super specialty teaching hospital which includes on site final disposal of BMW. Two types of costs are needed to be incurred by hospitals for BMW mgt, internal and external. Internal cost is the cost for segregation, mutilation, disinfection, internal storage and transportation including hidden cost of protective equipment. External cost involves off site transport of waste, treatment and final disposal.

COMMON REGIONAL FACILITY FOR FINAL DISPOSAL OF INFECTIOUS BMW

Hospitals, private practitioners, emergency care centres though aware of the rules do not have the time or resources to arrange satisfactory disposal of biomedical waste. Self contained on site treatment methods may be desirable and feasible for large healthcare facilities. They will not be practical or economical for smaller institutes. An acceptable common system should be in place which will provide free supply of colour coded bags, daily collection of infectious waste, safe transportation of waste to off site treatment facility and final disposal with suitable technology.

General waste like garbage, garden refuse etc. should join the stream of domestic refuse. Sharps should be collected in puncture proof containers. Bags and containers for infectious waste should be marked with Biohazard symbol. Highly infectious waste should be sterilised by autoclaving. Cytotoxic wastes are to be collected in leak proof containers clearly labelled as cytotoxic waste.

Needles and syringes should be destroyed with the help of needle destroyer and syringe cutters provided at the point of generation. Infusion sets, bottles and gloves should be cut with curved scissors. On site collection requires staff to close the waste bags when they are three quarters full either by tying the neck or by sealing the bag. Kerb side storage area needs to be impermeable and hard standing with good drainage. It should provide an easy access to waste collection vehicle.

Biomedical waste should be transported within the hospital by means of wheeled trolleys, containers or carts that are not used for any other intention. The trolleys have to be cleaned daily. Off site transportation vehicle should be marked with the name and address of carrier. Biohazard symbol should be painted. Suitable system for securing the load during transport should be ensured. Such a vehicle should be easily cleanable with rounded corners. All disposable plastic should be subjected to shredding before disposing off to vendor. Final treatment of biomedical waste can be done by technologies like etc.

REFERENCES

Benner, P. (1984). From novice to expert: Excellence and power in clinical nursing practice. Menlo Park, CA: Addison-Wesley.

Benner, P., & Wrubel, J. (1989). The primacy of caring. Menlo Park, CA: Addison–Wesley.

Diers, D. (1986). To profess—To be a professional. Journal of Nursing Administration, 16, 27.

Forbes, S. B. (1994). Hope: An essential human need in the elderly. Journal of Gerontological Nursing, 20(6), 5–10.

Isenalumhe, A. E. (2000). Using therapeutic support: My hands-on experience as a psychiatric nurse.

Locsin, R. C. (1998). Technologic competence as caring in critical care nursing. Holistic Nursing Practice, 12(4), 50–56.

Nightingale, F. (1969). Notes on nursing: What it is and what it is not. New York: Dover.

Peplau, H. (1952). Interpersonal relations in nursing. New York: Putnam.

Watson, J. (1988). Nursing: Human science and human care. New York: National League for Nursing.

Watson, J. (1999). Nursing: Human science and human care: A theory of nursing. Boston: Jones & Bartlett.

Watson, J. & Dossey, B. M. (1999). Postmodern nursing: Redefining nursing for the 21st century. London: Churchill Livingstone, Inc.

11

Medication Administration

The administration of medication is often a chief duty of the nurse. The practice of administering medication involves providing the patient with a substance prescribed and intended for the diagnosis, treatment, or prevention of a medical illness or condition.

GENERAL PRINCIPLES

The central action of medication administration involves actual and complete conveyance of a medication to the patient. However, there is a wider set of practices needed to achieve safe, effective patient outcomes and to prepare for and evaluate the outcome of medication administration.

Preparation for medication administration begins with the order for medication, in most circumstances written by the physician. Nurse practitioners and physician assistants are also often authorized to write prescriptions. State laws vary regarding these privileges. A record of orders for medication and other treatments is kept in the medical chart. Universally accepted safe clinical practice rules and state laws govern the components of medication orders in order to ensure consistency and patient safety. All orders should contain the patient's name, the date and time when the order is written, and the signature of the ordering clinician. Caregivers administering medication are accountable for checking that these components are present and clear. The name of the medication is accompanied by the dosage, or how much of the drug should be given; the route of administration, or how the medication should be given (i.e., intramuscular injection); and frequency, or how often the drug is to be given.

Many abbreviations are used in writing medication orders. Other common abbreviations include:

- p.o.: by mouth
- IM: intramuscular injection

- SC: subcutaneous injection
- IV: intravenous
- PR: per rectum
- h.s.: at hour of sleep (bedtime)
- ac: before meals
- pc: after meals
- q: every, ie, q 8 h means every 8 hours
- q.d.: every day
- b.i.d.: twice/day
- t.i.d.: three times/day
- q.i.d.: four times/day
- q.o.d.: every other day

Some examples of medication orders using these abbreviations are:

- digoxin 0.25 mg p.o. q.d.
- diphenhydramine 25 mg p.o. q h.s. prn.

If orders are illegible, ambiguous, or confusing, the author of the order should be consulted to clarify the order before any medication administration occurs. When the order is clear, it often needs to be transcribed to another document reserved for recording administration of medications. Health care institutions have specific policies regarding methods with which to check medication orders and ensure proper transcription. Policies also dictate parameters for order renewal or medication discontinuation.

Poor penmanship, misunderstanding of penmanship, and mistakes in transcription often contribute to medication mistakes. It is increasingly common for medical facilities to use a computerized system that lowers the risk of mistake by reducing steps in the process and validating information automatically.

Due to the large number of medications available and the large body of information needed for appropriate drug administration, it is significant to have access to a current medication reference such as the Physician's Desk Reference or other reference handbooks about medication. The package insert that comes with every medication is also a good resource. Pharmacists are knowledgeable resources and can answer many questions regarding medication. It is significant to be familiar with the medication ordered before attempting to administer it. Procedural manuals by the institution or medical reference publishers detail the step-by-step techniques for administering various types of medication.

FIVE RIGHTS

The patient should be notified of the order for the drug and provided with education about the medication they are to receive. Before administration, five factors often referred to as the "five rights" should be addressed. Medication records should be on hand at time of administration to ensure safe administration.

Right patient: Identify patient by name badge or bracelet. Avoid simply asking patient's name or checking the name on the door as miscommunications can sometimes occur.

Right drug: Check record for name of drug and compare with drug on hand. As many drugs have similar spellings, this needs to be checked carefully. For prevention of mistake, it is often recommended that three checks of the drug to be administered are made: when reaching for the package that contains the drug, when opening the drug, and when returning the packaging to its storage area. It is also recommended that clinicians only administer drugs that they have prepared, versus those prepared by another clinician.

Right route: Check medication record for how to administer the drug and check Labelling of drug to ensure it matches prescribed route.

Right dose: Compare ordered dose to dose on hand. At times, calculations may need to be performed to ascertain the correct dose. For instance, a scored tablet, or one that is designed and intended for dividing, may need to be halved or quartered in order to administer the correct oral dose. All medications should be handled to ensure that they do not come into contact with potentially contaminated objects or surfaces. Medications of any sort should not be left unattended, and patients should be observed taking the medication. This avoids the disposal, hoarding, abuse, or misuse of the medication, and assures the safety of the patient.

Documentation of medication administration is a significant duty. The medication record tells the story of what substances the patient has received and when. Like other health care records, it is also a legal document. Various institutions have policies and procedures regarding documentation. The initials of the administering nurse or other health care provider and the time and date should be documented on the record next to the appropriate order. Other information may be needed, such as location and severity of pain when administering a pain medicine (analgesic) or pulse rate when administering certain heart medications (i.e., digoxin). Patient refusals of medication also need to be documented, and the prescribing clinician should be informed.

Medication mistakes need to be documented as well. The prescribing clinician should be notified of mistakes. Institutional policies commonly require filing a separate form to document mistakes. Mistakes can include administering the wrong drug, wrong dose, at the wrong time, or via the wrong route. Omissions of medication are also considered mistakes.

It is significant to evaluate the patient following medication administration and document effect. For instance, many hospitals dictate that a note be written regarding pain relief within several hours after analgesic administration. Any adverse effects from medication should be reported.

DRUG PRESCRIPTION

The health care practitioner prescribes medications in different ways, depending on their purpose. Medications can be prescribed as stat, single-dose, standing, and prn orders.

STAT ORDERS

When the health care practitioner writes orders, the nurse should read all of the orders to determine if any stat orders have been prescribed. A stat order is an order for a single dose of medication to be given immediately. Stat drugs are often prescribed in emergency situations to modify a serious physiological response; a stat dose of nitro-glycerine may be ordered for a client experiencing chest pain. The nurse should assess and document the client's response to all stat medications.

SINGLE-DOSE ORDERS

Single-dose orders are one-time medications or may require the administration of drops or tablets over a short period of time. The nurse should administer single-dose orders only once, either at a time specified by the health care practitioner or at the earliest convenient time. These drugs are often prescribed in preparation for a diagnostic or therapeutic procedure; for example, radiopaque tablets may be administered in preparation for a gallbladder test, or a one-time order may be given for a preoperative medication.

STANDING ORDERS

Standing orders are also referred to as scheduled orders because they are administered routinely as specified until the order is cancelled by another order. The standing orders stay in effect until the health care practitioner discontinues or modifies the dosage or frequency with another order or until a prescribed number of days has elapsed as determined by agency policy. The purpose of a standing medication order is to maintain the desired blood level of the medication.

Agency policy determines the actual times for administering medications for a 24-hour time interval. For example, t.i.d. drugs may be administered at 0800, 1400, and 2000 or at 0900, 1500, and 2100. Medications ordered qd may have a specified time identified in the order, such as Isophane (NPH) Insulin 10 U SC qd at 0600, or they may be given at the agency's designated time, for example, Lanoxin 0.25 mg PO qd 0900. When the order specifies the number of days or the number of dosages of the drug the client is to receive, the order has an automatic stop date to discontinue the drug. For example, the order may read tetracycline 250 mg PO q6h for 5 days. The nurse should execute this order by administering 250 mg tetracycline orally every 6 hours for 5 days for a total of 20 doses. Day one begins with the administration of the drug and the time the first dose is given. If the first dose of tetracycline is given on a Tuesday at 1200, then every 6 hours, the last dose will be given on Sunday at 0600. Although the medication is given over 6 consecutive days, it totals 20 doses as ordered. Most agencies have an automatic stop date to discontinue certain medications, such as 5 or 7 days for antibiotics and 48 or 72 hours for narcotics.

PRN ORDERS

A drug may be ordered on a PRN (as needed) basis as circumstances indicate. The drug is administered when, in the nurse's judgment, the client's condition requires it. Before administering a PRN medication, the nurse must thoroughly assess the client, using both objective and subjective data in determining the appropriateness of administering the medication. This type of order is commonly written for analgesics, antiemetics, and laxatives. The order written by the health care practitioner indicates how frequently a PRN medication can be given.

A nurse cannot administer a PRN medication more frequently than the order indicates without consulting with the health care practitioner for a change in that order. Examples of PRN orders are meperidine (a narcotic analgesic) 75 mg IM q3-4 hours PRN incisional pain and Tylenol 650 mg q4 hours PRN headache. When the PRN medication has been administered, the nurse documents the assessment and the time of administration. In addition, the nurse is responsible for monitoring the effectiveness of the medication and documenting the effect in the client's medical record. The nurse administers the pain medication on the basis of the assessment of the client's pain and as specified in the order.

PARTS OF THE DRUG ORDER

All orders should be written clearly and legibly, and the drug order should contain seven parts:

- The name of the client
- The date and time when the order is written
- The name of the drug to be administered
- The dosage
- The route by which it is to be administered and special directives about its administration
- The time of administration and frequency
- The signature of the person writing the order, such as the physician or advanced practice registered nurse Drug prescriptions written in settings other than acute care facilities may also specify whether the generic or trade name of the drug is to be dispensed, the quantity to be dispensed, and how many times the prescription can be refilled.

ROUTES OF ADMINISTRATION

In pharmacology and toxicology, a route of administration is the path by which a drug, fluid, poison or other substance is brought into contact with the body.

A substance must be transported from the site of entry to the part of the body where its action is desired to take place (even if this only means penetration through the stratum corneum into the skin). However, using the body's transport mechanisms for this intention can be far from trivial. The pharmacokinetic properties of a drug (that is, those related to processes of uptake, distribution, and elimination) are critically determined by the route of administration.

CLASSIFICATION

Routes of administration can broadly be divided into:

- Topical: local effect, substance is applied directly where its action is desired.
- Enteral: desired effect is systemic (non-local), substance is given via the digestive tract.

- Parenteral: desired effect is systemic, substance is given by routes other than the digestive tract.

The following is a list of some routes of administration:

ORAL DRUGS ADMINISTRATION

Oral medication administration is the process by which drugs are delivered by mouth through the alimentary tract. Drugs are taken by this route because of convenience, absorption of the drug, ease of use, and cost containment. It is, hence, the most common method used.

Other routes are used when an individual cannot take anything by mouth, or the drug is poorly absorbed by the gastrointestinal tract. The nurse should check whether the patient has any known allergies. It is useful to remember the following checks when administering any medication: the right patient, the right medicine, the right route, the right dose, the right site, and the right time. Oral drugs are can be prescribed to be taken at different intervals, either before or after food. They can be in either liquid or solid form. Questions about the frequency with which drugs should be taken should be addressed to the primary health care provider.

Administration of oral medication should result in the patient receiving the proper dose of drug safely, and with no complications. Oral drugs can also interact with other medications that the patient is taking, such as injections. The nurse should check for any adverse reactions if the drug is being administered for the first time.

The staff should establish whether a patient is taking any drugs prior to being given any additional medication. It is significant that a nurse understand the actions, side effects, and incompatibility of drugs, recognize normal doses, and be knowledgeable about any reactions that a patient may experience. The nurse should report any unusual effects to the medical staff and record any side effects or negative reactions to the drug that has been given.

If the medication is to be prescribed regularly for a specific disease, the patient can be directed to a self-help group in which members have the same medical condition. The patient should be helped to feel confident that his or her privacy is ensured. If the labels on liquid medicine bottles are stained and illegible, the medicine should not be used.

PARENTERAL

When patients cannot use their gastrointestinal tracts for nutrition, parenteral nutrition may be used to maintain or improve the patient's nutritional status. This form of intravenous treatment provides all the nutrients that are delivered to the patient. This treatment may be temporary or long-term.

The harmful effects of malnutrition on the overall health of a patient are well documented. Poor nutrition is associated with slowed or impaired recovery from illness and surgery. For wound healing, tissue maintenance, and faster recovery, patients need optimal nutritional intake. When a patient is unable to take in enough food on his own, there are two options. Enteral feeding is preferred because it is less invasive, has a lower risk for infection, and is safer than the parenteral method. Though enteral feeding is the preferred route of nutritional intake, parenteral nutrition plays a significant role in many clinical situations. Patients who cannot consume enough nutrients on their own, or who cannot eat at all because of an illness, surgery, or an accident, may be fed through an intravenous line.

Patients receiving parenteral nutrition need to be monitored closely to ensure that the therapy is providing adequate amounts of fluids, minerals, and other nutrients that are required. Laboratory testing will take place on a regular basis to monitor the patient's status.

TOPICAL ADMINISTRATION

Vaginal medicines are topical agents prepared specifically for insertion into a woman's vagina. They are compounded in the form of a cream, foam, gel, tablet, or suppository, and are absorbed through the vaginal mucosa. Vaginal medicine in the form of a cream, foam, gel, or tablet is administered using a specific applicator that is provided by the manufacturer. Suppositories have the medicine suspended in wax and are shaped like a small bullet. They are inserted into the vagina with the index finger. Vaginal medicines are most often administered at bedtime, as the reclined position develops medication absorption. Vaginal medicines are most usually used to combat infection, inflammation, or dryness of the vaginal mucous. Other types of vaginal medicines include spermicides (i.e., to prevent conception), chaemotherapy (i.e., for cancer treatment), and aborticides (i.e., for inducing labour).

Vaginal tissue can be traumatized by the forceful use of applicators or fingernails during medicine administration, so medications should be introduced into the vagina gently. Patients should be encouraged to relax, as this will decrease resistance to the mode of insertion. One should not attempt to insert vaginal medication when a patient is confused and combative. Medicine should not be delivered via the vagina if it is not labelled for vaginal use. Vaginal medicine should not be taken orally.

A female staff member must be present in the room when a male nurse administers a vaginal medication. The patient should be positioned on her back, with knees bent. Her legs should be drawn up toward the hips, and the heels should be flat on the bed. A sheet across the abdomen and upper legs, falling just over the knees, will decrease the patient's feeling of exposure. Directions for filling the applicator should followed. At this point, the patient should be advised to drop her knees apart. The nurse should wash his or her hands and put on disposable gloves. Using one hand, the nurse should spread the labia and expose the vaginal opening. If there is drainage or exudate, the nurse should cleanse the area with warm, soapy water, using cotton balls or a clean washcloth. The vaginal opening should be rinsed and allowed to air dry. A small amount of water-soluble lubricant should then be placed on the tip of the applicator or suppository, the labia spread, and the suppository or applicator tipped into the vaginal opening. The suppository or applicator should be moved gently down, toward the posterior (i.e., back) wall of the vagina, toward the spine 2-4 inches (5-10 cm), or until resistance is felt. The suppository or applicator should then be angled upward. When using an applicator to deliver cream or gel, the plunger should be gently pushed to deliver the medicine. The nurse should then remove his or her finger and/or the applicator from the vagina. The disposable latex gloves should be disposed of correctly.

Before beginning to administer vaginal medicines, the door to the room should be closed to ensure privacy. (A female staff member must already be present if the nurse is a male.) The patient should empty her bladder just before administration. The nurse should check the medication label each time medicine is given; this will avoid medication mistakes. The medication must be checked to confirm that it is the right medicine, the right dose (i.e., strength), the right time, the right patient, and the right method of administration. The expiration date on the label should be checked; outdated medication should never be used. If the nurse has not yet put on disposable gloves, it should be done at this time. His or her hands should be washed, and gloves should be put on.

The used applicator should be placed on a clean paper towel to prevent the spread of micro-organisma. The patient should be covered and encouraged to maintain a reclined position, with knees up, for at least 10 minutes (30 minutes after a suppository). This will allow time for medicine absorption. If the applicator is reusable, it should be washed in warm soapy water, thoroughly rinsed, air dried, and placed back in the medicine box or a plastic bag until the next use. The used gloves and disposable applicator should be put into a trash bag, which can be sealed and discarded. The nurse should wash his or her hands. The patient should be given a mini-pad (or small sanitary napkins) to protect her underwear from medicine that may leak out.

The patient should not instructed not to use tampons after vaginal medicine administration; they will absorb the medicine more rapidly than the vaginal mucosa, and the full effect of the drug will not be achieved.

Tissue irritation or allergic reactions can result from vaginal medications. If irritation, swelling, or redness of the tissue is apparent, or if the patient complains of pain or burning, the next dose of medicine should not be given until the physician has been consulted.

Most vaginal medicines will produce the desired effects within several days to one week. Spermicides and aborticide vaginal medicines act more rapidly when used as directed. If the client experiences vaginal pain at the time of medicine instillation, or the condition does not improve, the physician should be contacted.

Vaginal medicines are administered by a licensed nurse (i.e., R.N. or L.P.N.) in the health care setting. An alert and cooperative patient may be allowed to administer the medicine under the direction of the nurse. The nurse should, nevertheless, evaluate the site and the effectiveness of the medicine. The patient, or members of the patient's family, can be taught to administer vaginal medicines in the home setting.

RECTAL

Rectal medicines are medications prepared specifically for insertion into the rectum. They are compounded in many forms. Liquid rectal medicine solutions are given by enema. Creams, lotions and ointments are applied externally or inserted internally using an applicator. Suppositories are prepared by mixing medicine with a wax-like substance to form a semi-solid, bullet-shaped form that will melt after insertion into the rectum.

Rectal medications are administered for a localized effect on the rectum or for a systemic effect when a patient is vomiting, unable to swallow, or unconscious. Rectal medicine is most usually used as a localized treatment for constipation or as a topical treatment for rectal inflammation or infection. Rectal suppositories may be used for the treatment of fever, nausea, and pain; they may also be prescribed to induce sedation or bronchodilation, or to reduce the nausea and vomiting that can accompany chaemotherapy. Medicated enemas may be used to cleanse the bowel, to combat bacteria, or to kill parasites.

Rectal medications must be used with caution in the cardiac patient who has arrhythmias or has recently had a myocardial infarction (i.e., heart attack). Insertion of a rectal medicine can cause vagus nerve stimulation and may trigger an arrhythmia-such as bradycardia. Rectal medicines should not be given to the patient with undiagnosed abdominal pain because peristalsis of the bowel can cause an inflamed appendix to rupture. Rectal medicines should be used cautiously in patients who have undergone recent surgery on the rectum, bowel, or prostate gland. If the patient has rectal bleeding or a prolapse of rectal tissue from the rectal opening, the medicine should be withheld and the physician consulted before administration. Rectal medicines should not be taken orally, and only medications labelled as rectal preparations should be placed in the rectum.

Administration of rectal medication should be done after the patient is positioned properly. Lifting the upper buttocks will enable visualization of his or her rectal opening. External lotions, ointments or creams can be applied directly, using a gloved finger or a 4×4 gauze pad. Prior to administering internal rectal medicine, the tip of the suppository, enema catheter, or applicator should be lubricated with a water-soluble lubricant. To insert a rectal suppository, the lubricated, tapered end of the suppository should be placed at the rectal opening and gently pushed into the rectum. The suppository should be pushed continuously toward the umbilicus until the full length of the nurse's gloved index finger has been inserted into the rectal opening (i.e., about 3 inches, or7.5 cm, for an adult patient). When inserting suppositories into children, the suppository should be pushed about 1 inch (2.5 cm) beyond the rectal opening, or up to the first knuckle of the nurse's index finger. When inserting suppositories into infants, the little finger should be inserted one-half inch (1.25 cm) beyond the rectal opening. The buttocks should be released and the finger removed.

When given properly, rectal medications work within 30-60 minutes to relieve pain, nausea, constipation, or fever. Rectal ointments for swelling and irritation of haemorrhoids may reverse the condition within several days. Because of their liquid state, rectal enemas are absorbed quickly and work rapidly. Retention enemas are meant to be held for 30 minutes to achieve full therapeutic effect.

Rectal medicines are administered by a licensed nurse (R.N. or L.P.N.) in the health care setting. An alert and cooperative patient may be allowed to apply external and internal rectal ointments and suppositories under the direction of the nurse. The nurse, nevertheless, should evaluate the site and the effectiveness of the medicine. The patient or members of the patient's family can be taught to administer rectal medicines in the home setting.

EAR INSTILLATION

An ear instillation is a solution of topical medicine prepared for administration into the ear canal. Medicine instilled into the ear is absorbed through the skin of the ear canal and membranes of the eardrum. Ear instillations are used primarily to treat wax build-up and inflammations or infections of the ear.

Do not place the medicine dropper tip or cotton swabs directly into the ear canal, as this can traumatize the skin of the ear canal. Do not touch anything with the tip of the medicine dropper to prevent contamination. If the patient experiences pain from eardrops, stop using the medicine and contact the physician. To instil eardrops, have the patient lie on his or her side with the affected ear up. Gently pull the lobe of the ear up and back to open the ear canal (down and back for children under the age of three). Hold the medicine dropper just above the entrance to the ear canal and squeeze out the correct number of drops. Release the ear and have the patient remain still for five minutes to allow absorption of the eardrops. Repeat the procedure on the other ear if ordered.

The hands should be washed before administering ear drops. Check the medication label each time to avoid medication mistakes. Be sure it is the right medicine, the right dose (strength), the right time, the right individual and the right method. Look at the expiration date on the label. Do not use outdated medicine. Warm the eardrops to body temperature by rolling the bottle in the hands for several minutes before the instillation. Have tissues or a warm washcloth available to wipe off residual medicine that may drip out of the ear when the patient sits up. A small piece of clean cotton ball may be placed into the outer portion of the ear canal to absorb excess medicine if desired. Discard soiled tissues and cotton in a bag that can be closed and discarded. Wipe the tip of the ear dropper with a clean tissue and recap the bottle. The hands should be washed again after completing the procedure. Excessive use of eardrops can cause irritation and inflammation of the skin and membranes of the ear.

Ear instillations will produce the desired results within a few days. Contact the physician if the patient experiences ear pain at the time of medicine instillation, or if the condition does not improve. Ear instillations are commonly administered by a licensed nurse (R.N. or L.P.N.) in the health care setting. The patient or members of the patient's family can be taught to instil ear medicines in the home setting.

INHALATION

Inhalation (also known as inspiration) is the movement of air from the external environment, through the air ways, and into the alveoli.

Inhalation begins with the onset of contraction of the diaphragm, which results in expansion of the intrapleural space and an increase in negative pressure according to Boyle's Law. This negative pressure generates airflow because of the pressure difference between the atmosphere and alveolus. Air enters, inflating the lung through either the nose or the mouth into the pharynx (throat) and trachea before entering the alveoli.

A nasal inhalation system is provided for vaporizing a selected medicament or the like and for convenient inhalation of the resultant vapours. In one form, the inhalation system comprises a nozzle mounted at the discharge end of a source of air flow, preferably a heated air flow, wherein the nozzle is shaped to support a medicament-containing inhaler tube for flow-through passage of the air flow to produce medicinal vapours. A conveniently sterilizable vented adapter sleeve may be carried about the inhaler tube and/or mounted on the nozzle to prevent human contact with the inhaler tube and to limit the quantitative air flow to a person's nostrils. In an alternative form, a plurality of inhaler tubes are supported within a turret assembly mounted at the discharge end of the air flow source and rotatable to align a selected one of the inhaler tubes with an open discharge tube thereby permitting flow-through passage of air.

RECORDING AND REPORTING OF MEDICATIONS ADMINISTERED

Monitoring and measuring mistakes in health care present any challenges. Traditionally, many clinicians have hesitated to report mistakes for fear of punishment or sanction. Some health care workers may avoid reporting mistakes made by other clinicians out of concern that filing a report would get someone in "trouble." Though clinicians always have been concerned about safety, it has not been clear how reporting mistakes could lead to clinical improvements or mistake reduction.

Many health care facilities have implemented some type of variance or occurrence reporting system in an effort to track adverse events or unusual occurrences. Rarely do systems such as these track "near misses" or minor mistakes that do not result in patient injury. Regardless of the type of monitoring system, the value of consistently reporting and recording all types of mistakes or near misses has not been made clear to clinicians or administrators. Even when data are collected, they are not used consistently or systematically to examine factors that contribute to mistakes.

In many hospitals, for instance, incident reports related to medication mistakes are placed in a clinician's personnel file to track his or her personal mistake rate. No one systematically examines and analyzes these reports to identify trends. To understand mistakes of any type, trends and factors that contribute to mistakes must be identified. In the case of medication mistakes, it would be helpful to know whether they occur on a specific clinical unit or shift or at a specific service or time of day. Also, it would be helpful to know whether similarities exist among mistakes related to the providers who wrote medication orders, the pharmacists who dispensed medications, the patients' acuity, or the types of medications. Monitoring and recording this type of data would provide helpful information that could be used to minimize subsequent mistakes. Currently, this information is not readily available, and if it has been collected, it may not be reliable, valid, or amenable to interpretation.

STORAGE AND MAINTENANCE OF DRUGS

Drugs are dispensed by the pharmacy to nursing units through various methods to accommodate the agency's medication system. Once the pharmacy delivers the drugs to a nursing unit, the nurse is responsible for their safe storage. Scheduled drugs for each client are usually dispensed in a unit-dose form. Unit dose is a system of packaging and Labelling each dose of medication by pharmacy, often to supply a 24-hour time period. The pharmacy usually delivers the drugs and stores the drugs in the designated area for each client. Unit-dose drugs are usually stored in a medication cart that contains individual drawers for each client's medication supply or in the medication room in a separate, organized container for each client. The unit-dose system has made it easier for nurses to administer the correct dose, thereby reducing the number of medication errors.

The nurse, usually at the beginning of each shift, checks the medications in each client's drawer. Some medications carts are locked, and the nurse keeps the key. Medication drawers should be removed only one at a time from the cart when the nurse is preparing the medication for administration. The client's drawer should never be left unattended on top of the cart. Drugs should not be removed from one client's supply for administration to another client. Certain drugs are stock supplied (dispensed and labelled in large quantities) and stored in the medication room or other area on the nursing unit. Stock supplies are kept together in a secured area. Certain intravenous fluids and medications must be stored in the medication refrigerator to preserve the integrity of the drug. The Public Health Department and accrediting agencies mandate that only drugs can be stored in the medication refrigerator.

NARCOTICS AND CONTROLLED SUBSTANCES

Health care agencies have forms to record the supply on hand and the administration of narcotics and controlled substances in accord with federal regulations. These forms usually require the recording of the following information for each drug administered:

- Amount of the drug used
- Name of the client receiving the drug
- Name of the nurse administering the drug
- Name of the prescribing health care practitioner
- Time the drug was administered

Nursing practice usually requires that nurses count the narcotics and controlled substances at specified intervals. For example, at the change of shifts, one nurse who is going off duty counts the drugs with a nurse coming on duty. Each drug used must be accounted for on the narcotic record. When the narcotic count does not check, the nurse must report the discrepancy immediately. Narcotics and controlled substances are kept in a doublelocked drawer, box, room, or medication-dispensing cart. The law requires these safety precautions in the use of narcotics and controlled substances to aid in the control of drug misuse. If for any reason a narcotic has to be discarded, a second person should act as a witness and that person should also sign the narcotic sheet.

REFERENCES

Bottorff, J., & Morse, J. (1994). Identifying types of attending: Patterns of nurses' work. Image, 26(1), 53.

Cochrane, D., & Oberle, K. (1992, July). Do they really understand us? American Journal of Nursing, 92(7), 20.

Edelman, C. L., & Mandle, C. L. (1997). Health promotion throughout the lifespan (4th ed.). St. Louis: Mosby.

Giger, J. N., & Davidhizar, R. E. (1999). Transcultural nursing: Assessment and intervention (3rd ed.) (pp. 43–60). St. Louis: Mosby.

Hubert, P. M. (1998). Revealing patient concerns. American Journal of Nursing, 98(10), 16H–16L.

Johnson, B. S. (1996). Psychiatric-mental health nursing: Adaptation and growth (4th ed.). Philadelphia: Lippincott.

Kneisl, C. R. (1996). Therapeutic communication. In H. S. Wilson & C. R. Kneisl (Eds.), Psychiatric nursing (5th ed.). Menlo Park, CA: Addison-Wesley.

Masching, J. (1996). A nurse battling with her own depression. Journal of Psychosocial Nursing, 34(9), 26–29.

Olen, D. R. (1993). Communicating. Milwaukee: JODA Communications.

Peplau, H. (1960). Talking with patients. American Journal of Nursing, 60(7), 964.

Varcarolis, E., & Rader, I. (1998). Foundations of mental health-psychiatric nursing (3rd ed.). Philadelphia: Saunders.

Ward-Collins, D. (1998). "Noncompliant." Isn't there a better way to say it? American Journal of Nursing, 98(5), 27–31.

12

Perioperative Patients

Perioperative refers to the total span of surgical intervention. Surgical intervention is a common treatment for injury, disease, or disorder. The surgeon intervenes in the disease process by repairing, removing, or replacing body tissues or organs. Surgery is invasive because an incision is made into the body or a part of the body is removed.

Effective perioperative management is directed by a multidisciplinary team in accordance with recognized standards of care and individualized expected client outcomes. Institutional protocol, which defines how procedures will be performed, is initiated in the preoperative phase and continues throughout the other phases. Each member of the health care team (surgeon, anaesthetist, and nurse) has a specific role and responsibility toward the perioperative client. Collaboration between all health care providers is essential in planning client care. "Collaboration means that people with different areas of expertise are working as equals to define issues, design solutions, and achieve high quality outcome".

CONCEPT OF PERIOPERATIVE NURSING

Perioperative patient care is a variety of nursing activities carried out before, during, and after surgery. The perioperative period has three phases:

- The preoperative phase begins with the decision that surgical intervention is necessary and ends when the patient is transferred to the operating room table.
- The intraoperative phase is the period during which the patient is undergoing surgery in the operating room. It ends when the patient is transferred to the post-anaesthesia recovery room.

- The postoperative phase lasts from the patient's admission to the recovery room through the complete recovery from surgery.

PREOPERATIVE PHASE

The primary goal of preoperative nursing care is to place the client in the best possible condition for surgery through careful assessment and thorough preparation. Assessment of the client's status before surgery establishes baseline data to direct interventions throughout the perioperative phases. Each member of the health care team has identified functions relating to the assessment of the client's physiological, psychological, social, cultural, and spiritual status. The findings from the client's assessment must be documented throughout the surgical experience. Assessment of the perioperative client includes a nursing history and physical examination.

A complete assessment is performed on the outpatient client during the preadmission visit. On the day of surgery, the nurse conducts a focused assessment to ensure current, accurate data. During the assessment process, the nurse evaluates the client's level of anxiety and fear. Anxiety is a vague, uneasy feeling whose source is often non-specific or unknown to the client. Fear is a feeling of dread related to an identifiable source that the client validates. Anxiety also has well-defined physiological changes, such as an increased heart rate, clammy hands, muscular tension (especially in the neck muscles), and behavioural manifestations, such as rapid speech and irritability.

PREPARATION OF PATIENT

The perioperative nursing history provides information relative to factors that can increase a client's risk or influence the expected surgical outcomes. Pertinent data are obtained from the client interview: medical history including family history of anaesthesia complications (malignant hypertension); medications; allergies; age related factors; social, cultural, and spiritual concerns; and psychological status. Nurses should conduct the interview in a quiet room, free from background noise. Many elderly clients have some degree of high-tone hearing loss, so it is necessary to speak in a strong, clear voice. Clients who have difficulty comprehending the surgical procedure should have a responsible family member present during the interview. A third person can help clarify precisely what the nurse said and can interpret such instructions to other family members.

Medical History

The nurse reviews the client's medical record. The surgeon's history and physical findings provide pertinent data regarding the reasons for surgery. If the client was previously hospitalized, the nurse obtains the previous medical records to have available on the nursing unit. Hospitalization records are reviewed to gain an overview of the client's health status because preexisting medical conditions can increase the client's surgical risks. During the interview, the nurse questions the client regarding past illnesses and the main reason for seeking surgical treatment. The client is asked to describe prior surgeries and their dates.

Any complications from a previous surgery or anaesthesia should be recorded. It is important to note if the client has had prior blood transfusions or reactions. At this time the nurse can ascertain whether the client has objections to receiving blood or blood products or has made arrangements for blood replacement. Some clients prefer to donate their own blood in advance so that it can be held in reserve if the need for it arises during surgery.

Family members or friends may also donate blood to decrease the cost to the client. During the nursing history, the nurse needs to assess exactly what drugs the client has been taking. The client's response to questions about the use of alcohol, tobacco, "street drugs," prescription, over-the-counter drugs, and herbs should be documented because these substances have surgical implications. Certain prescription drugs (antihypertensives, tranquilizers, steroids, and diuretics) can increase the client's anaesthesia risks.

Clients with chronic diseases are likely to be taking numerous medications that can cause complications during the perioperative period. The nurse assesses the client's physiological health status by performing either a partial or a complete physical examination. The decision to conduct a partial or complete physical depends on the client's health status relative to the surgical procedure, the setting, and the amount of time available to gather pertinent data. The nurse in an outpatient setting, on the day of surgery, usually performs a partial examination. The client's medical record should be reviewed to ensure that a complete nursing physical was conducted during the preadmission visit. The nurse should focus on obtaining pertinent assessment data to establish baseline parameters for prioritizing the client's care.

The client's neurological assessment is integrated throughout the interview and physical examination. Preparing the client for surgery requires the nurse to perform multiple interventions within specific time constraints. However, the nurse must remain responsive to the client's needs, demonstrating a caring attitude. Documentation tools are available to assist the nurse in providing safe, timely preoperative care (e.g., the consent form and preoperative checklist). Active planning and intervention are necessary to reduce the risk for complications.

Surgical Consent Form

Although surgeons are responsible for obtaining informed consent, nurses should verify that consent has been obtained before treatment begins. Consent is given only for the extent of action documented on the informed consent. Nurses can identify problems with consent when the client:

- Cannot explain the procedure or identify the risks
- Signed the form more than 30 days before surgery
- Had an unauthorized person sign the consent form
- Did not sign the consent form

The nurse should notify the surgeon in the event that any problems with consent are identified. If the surgeon proceeds without appropriate consent, nursing administration should be notified and the nurse should make personal notations outside the medical record. This practice protects the nurse should the situation be brought to court. If the client reverses a decision and decides against surgery, the nurse is obligated to inform the surgeon in order to prevent unwanted treatment.

Preoperative Checklist

A checklist is a form that allows the nurse to insert a checkmark (?) beside symptoms or to fill in one or two words in answer to a cue or a question. Although some variations exist in how agencies format the preoperative checklist, the forms usually have similar content. Nursing activities are usually designated by time intervals: "night before surgery" and "day of surgery." Time designations help to prevent surgical delays that can increase the client's anxiety and the agency's costs. This preparation ensures that assessment, diagnostic tests, and teaching were done on the preadmission visit and allows time to obtain missing information and to assess the need for reinforcement or reevaluation as necessary.

On the day of surgery, the nurse focuses on the immediate physical interventions to prepare the client for surgery. While admitting and preparing the client for surgery, the nurse uses this time to encourage the client to verbalize any concerns. Allowance should be made for family members or significant others to remain with the client as the client awaits transfer to the operating room.

INTRAOPERATIVE PHASE

The term "intraoperative" refers to the time during surgery. Intraoperative care is patient care during an operation and ancillary to that operation.

Activities such as monitoring the patient's vital signs, blood oxygenation levels, fluid therapy, medication transfusion, anaesthesia, radiography, and retrieving samples for laboratory tests, are examples of intraoperative care. Intraoperative care is provided by nurses, anaesthesiologists, nurse anaesthetists, surgical technicians, surgeons, and residents, all working as a team.

Intraoperative care includes the activities performed by the health care team during surgery that ensure the patient's safety and comfort, implement the surgical procedure, monitor and maintain vital functions, and document care given. The intraoperative time period can vary greatly from less than one hour to 12 hours or more, depending on the complexity of the surgery being performed.

Operation Theatre Set Up and Environment

The surgical area usually consists of three zones: unrestricted, semirestricted, and restricted. The unrestricted area is designed for personnel to enter in street clothes: receiving desk, holding area, and locker rooms. Surgical attire (scrub clothes, disposable shoe covers, and caps) is required in the semirestricted and restricted zones. Hallways and storage areas constitute the semirestricted area. Restricted zones (controlled and germ-free areas) include the OR and rooms where sterile instruments are prepared.

Holding Area

The holding area is a unit where the surgical team prepares the client for surgery. The anaesthetist usually starts the intravenous infusion and administers the preoperative intravenous medication. The nurse confirms that aspects of care on the preoperative checklist have been performed. A family member is usually encouraged to remain with the client while the client awaits transfer to the OR.

Surgical Team

The surgical team consists of the surgeon, anaesthetist, OR nurses, surgical assistants, and other members of the health care team. The roles and responsibilities of the surgeon and anaesthetist have already been discussed. The OR team usually consists of:

- Surgeon: Scrubbed and in surgical attire to perform the surgery
- Anaesthesia provider: Masked and in clean scrub attire to administer the anaesthesia
- Surgical assistant (first assistant): Can be another physician, a nurse, or physician's assistant (PA) who is scrubbed, in sterile attire, and assists the surgeon to ligate, suction, and suture
- Scrub nurse or technician: Scrubbed and in sterile attire; prepares the instrument tray and passes the instruments, sponges, needles, and sutures to the surgeon
- Circulating nurse: In clean scrub attire and mask; obtains supplies, delivers materials, pours solutions, handles specimens, positions the client and surgical drapes, and disposes of soiled items

Both the scrub and circulating nurses are responsible for counting the number of used instruments, needles, and sponges. Before the surgeon closes the incision, these items are counted to ensure that nothing is being left in the operative site.

Role of Nurse

The first activity of assessment for the OR nurse is to check the client's identification band and confirm the surgical site. Agency protocol and standards of care from the AORN establish the focus areas of assessment for the client and the environment. Assessment of proper positioning to ensure comfort and safety includes: o Checking for client alterations that can affect positioning during the procedure, such as previous skeletal or joint surgery, presence of a joint or vascular prothesis, poor nutrition, and skin integrity o Making sure the OR bed is prepared to receive the client: for example, warming mattress on bed, proper orientation of bed, bed wheels locked o Ensuring that accessories are clean and readily available for a specific position: for example, Wilson frame, chest rolls, pillows, headrest Throughout the surgical procedure, the nurse assesses for pressure areas of the extremities, joints, or any body surface; skin discolouration; and temperature. Whenever the client's position is changed during surgery, the nurse reassesses for signs of circulatory impairment from positioning and equipment in contact with the skin.

Common intraoperative nursing diagnoses promote client comfort, safety, and support during the surgical procedure. The focus of intraoperative care planning is on nursing activities that promote the client's achievement of expected intraoperative outcomes.

These outcomes are directed at placing the client in a safe environment free from injury. The OR team monitors the client throughout the surgical procedure for complications. Specific nursing care is planned to encompass the surgeon's specifications for positioning and to alleviate or prevent any individual client problem.

Surgeons have preference cards that identify the type of equipment and instruments for various surgical procedures (e.g., indications and use of electrical equipment). Planning also involves determining the appropriate mode of client transfer, determining equipment and positioning aids, or determining the need for ancillary personnel to accomplish These outcomes are directed at placing the client in a safe environment free from injury.

The OR team monitors the client throughout the surgical procedure for complications. Specific nursing care is planned to encompass the surgeon's specifications for positioning and to alleviate or prevent any individual client problem. Surgeons have preference cards that identify the type of equipment and instruments for various surgical procedures (e.g., indications and use of electrical equipment). Planning also involves determining the appropriate mode of client transfer, determining equipment and positioning aids, or determining the need for ancillary personnel to accomplish the positioning. The plan of care should be individualized to include needs relative to the client's health status such as diabetes, malnourishment, or paralysis.

Nursing interventions are selected to facilitate caring and to achieve the expected outcomes, such as the client is free from infection 72 hours postoperatively. Because anaesthesia inhibits the client's ability to protect self, the OR staff implements surgical asepsis, safe positioning, and other interventions that promote client safety (e.g., the client is never left unattended). Nursing care includes communication skills to reduce the client's anxiety. The OR staff communicates a caring attitude, functioning under the assumption that anaesthetized clients will be able to recall comments made during surgery.

POSTOPERATIVE PHASE

The time after surgery is referred to as the postoperative period and includes the recovery and convalescence phases. The recovery phase is the time immediately after surgery when the effects of anaesthesia are wearing off and the patient is waking up. The convalescence phase is spent either in the hospital, in an interim care facility, or at home-depending on the procedure and the preferences of the physician and patient.

Intraoperative complications are surgery related, anaesthesia related, or position related. One complication occurring during the intraoperative period that is not common but can be life threatening is an anaphylactic (allergic) reaction to anaesthesia. The intraoperative staff is trained extensively in the treatment of such a reaction, and emergency equipment should always be available in the event it is required for this intention. Another anaesthesia-related complication is called "awareness under anaesthesia." This occurs when the patient receives sufficient muscle relaxant (paralytic agent) to prohibit voluntary motor function but insufficient sedation and analgesia to block pain and the sense of hearing. Patients are aware of being "awake" because they hear the sounds and conversation in the room and, in some cases, can feel the pain associated with the skin incision and surgery. However, they cannot respond to these sensations in a way-not even with so small a motion as blinking the eyelid-that will tell someone what they are sensing. This condition creates an exaggerated fear response that can affect haemodynamics and vital signs. Another complicating reaction may be that of malignant hyperthermia. This is a chain reaction triggered in susceptible people by usually used general anaesthetics. Signs include greatly increased body metabolism, muscle rigidity, and eventual hyperthermia which may exceed 110°F (43.3°C). Death may be caused by cardiac arrest, brain damage, internal haemorrhage, or failure of other body systems.

Complications of surgery include, but are not limited to, hypovolemic shock (due to blood loss during surgery), injuries from poor positioning during surgery, infection of the surgical wound, fluid and electrolyte imbalances, aspiration pneumonia, blood clots, and paralytic ileus (paralysis of the intestines, causing distention).

Nurses may fill two different roles in the operating room. The scrub nurse is accountable for providing the surgeon with instruments and supplies and maintaining the sterile field. This role also may be assumed by a scrub or surgical technician. The second role nurses have in the operating room is that of circulating nurse. The circulating nurse is first the patient's advocate, with primary concern and duty for the patient's safety and welfare. In addition, the circulating nurse is accountable for anything related to the patient that is not directly contingent to the sterile field. That means all activities necessary to prepare the patient and the operative site for surgery, and assistance needed by anaesthesia personnel. Of crucial import is that the circulating nurse must be certified to give intravenous medication to the patient in case of an emergency. Finally, nurses must document and process tissue specimens for pathology.

WOUNDS

A wound occurs when the integrity of skin is compromised (e.g., skin breaks, burns, or bone fractures). A wound may be caused by an act, such as a gunshot, fall, or surgical procedure; by an infectious disease; or by an underlying condition.

TYPES & CLASSIFICATIONS

Types and causes of wounds are wide ranging. They may be chronic, as are pressure ulcers (which are common in persons with diabetes as a result of skin breakdown)-or they may be acute, as in gunshot wounds or an animal bites. Wounds may also be referred to as open, in which the skin has been compromised and underlying tissues are exposed. Alternatively, they may be closed. Here, the skin has not been compromised, but trauma to underlying tissue has occurred (e.g., a bruised rib or cerebral contusion). Emergency personnel generally place acute wounds in one of eight categories:

- Abrasions: Also called scrapes, they occur when the skin is rubbed away by friction against a rough surface (e.g., rope burns and skinned knees).
- Avulsions: Occur when an entire structure or part of it is forcibly pulled away, such as in the loss of a permanent tooth or an ear lobe. Explosions, gunshots, and animal bites may cause avulsions.
- Contusions: Also called bruises, these are the result of a forceful trauma that injures an internal structure without breaking the skin. Blows to the chest, abdomen, or head with a blunt instrument (e.g., a football or a fist) can cause contusions.
- Crush wounds: Occur when a heavy object falls onto a person, splitting the skin and shattering or tearing underlying structures.
- Cuts: These are slicing wounds made with a sharp instrument, leaving even edges, or those made with a dull cutting instrument,

which leaves uneven edges. Cuts may be as minimal as those caused by paper (i.e., paper cuts), or as significant as a surgical incisions.

- Lacerations: Also called tears, these are separating wounds that produce ragged edges. They are produced by a tremendous force against the body, either from an internal source, as in childbirth, or from an external source, like a punch.
- Missile wounds: Also called velocity wounds, they are caused by an object entering the body at a high speed, normally a bullet.
- Punctures: Deep, narrow wounds produced by sharp objects such as nails, knives, and broken glass.

WOUND HEALING PROCESS

Treatment of wounds involves stopping any bleeding, then cleaning and dressing the wound to prevent infection. Additional medical attention may be needed if the effects of the wound have compromised the body's ability to function effectively.

Stopping the Bleeding

Most bleeding may be stopped by direct pressure. Direct pressure is applied by placing a clean cloth or dressing over the wound and pressing the palm of the hand over the entire area. This limits local bleeding without disrupting a significant portion of the circulation. The cloth absorbs blood and allows clot formation. The clot should not be disturbed. Therefore, if blood soaks through the original cloth, another one should be placed directly on top of it. The new cloth should not be replace the original one.

If the wound is on an arm or a leg that does not appear to have a broken bone, the injured limb should be elevated to a height above the person's heart, while direct pressure is applied. Elevating the wound allows gravity to slow the flow of blood to that area.

If severe bleeding cannot be stopped by direct pressure or with elevation, the next step is to apply pressure to the major artery supplying blood to the area of the wound. In the arm, pressure would be applied to the brachial artery by pressing the inside of the upper arm against the bone. In the leg, pressure would be applied to the femoral artery by pressing on the inner crease of the groin, against the pelvic bone.

If the bleeding from an arm or leg is so extreme as to be life threatening, and if it cannot be stopped by any other means, a tourniquet may be needed. However, in the process of limiting further blood loss, the tourniquet also drastically deprives the limb tissues of oxygen. As a result, the patient may live, but the limb may die.

Dressing the Wound

Once the bleeding has been stopped, cleaning and dressing the wound is significant for preventing infection. Though the flowing blood flushes debris from the wound, running water should also be used to rinse away dirt. Embedded particles, such as wood slivers and glass splinters-if not too deep-may be removed with a needle or pair of tweezers that has been sterilized in rubbing alcohol or in the heat of a flame. Once the wound has been cleared of foreign material and washed, it should be blotted dry gently, with care not to disturb the blood clot. An antibiotic ointment may be applied. The wound should then be covered with a clean dressing and a bandage to hold the dressing in place. Depending on the wound type, dressings can be designed to retain (or absorb) moisture, or to rehydrate desiccated wounds. Dressing materials may include polyurethane films or foams, hydrogels, hydrofibre, calcium alginates, and hydrocolloids.

Getting Medical Assistance

An individual who has become impaled on a fixed object, such as a fence post or a stake in the ground, should only be moved by emergency medical personnel. Foreign objects embedded in the eye should only be removed by a physician. Larger penetrating objects, such as a fishhook or an arrow, should only be removed by a doctor, who can prevent further damage as the object is extracted.

In several instances, additional medical attention will be necessary. Wounds that penetrate the muscle beneath the skin should be cleaned and treated by a doctor, and may require stitches to stay closed during healing. Some deep wounds that do not extend to the underlying muscle may only require butterfly bandages. Wounds to the face and neck, even small ones, should always be examined by a physician so that scarring can be minimized and sensory function can be preserved. Deep wounds to the hands and wrists should be examined for nerve and tendon damage. Puncture wounds may require a tetanus shot to prevent serious infection. Animal bites should always be examined and the possibility of rabies infection considered.

Infection

Wounds that develop signs of infection should also be brought to a doctor's attention. Signs of infection arc swelling, redness, tenderness, throbbing pain, localized warmth, fever, swollen lymph glands, the presence of pus either in the wound or draining from it, and red streaks spreading away from the wound.

Emergency Treatment

With as little as one quart of blood lost, an individual may lose consciousness and go into traumatic shock. If the individual stops breathing, artificial respiration should be administered. In the absence of a pulse, cardiopulmonary resuscitation (CPR) must be performed. Once the individual is breathing unassisted, one can attend to the bleeding.

In cases of severe blood loss, treatment may include the intravenous replacement of body fluids. This may be infusion with saline or plasma, or with a whole-blood transfusion.

Some alternative therapies may help to support the injured individual. Homeopathic remedies include: Ledum (Ledum palustre) taken internally for puncture wounds, calendula (Calendula officinalis) or tea tree oil (Melaleuca spp.) used topically as an antiseptic, aloe (Aloe barbadensis) applied topically to soothe skin during healing, and St. John's wort (Hypericum perforatum) used internally or topically when wounds affect the nerves, especially in the arms and legs. Acupuncture is thought to support the healing process by restoring energy flow in the meridians affected by the wound. In some cases, vitamin E, taken orally or applied topically, may speed healing and prevent scarring.

COMPLICATIONS OF WOUND HEALING

Following are the complications of wound healing:

- Haematoma: dressings should be inspected for haemorrhage at intervals during the first 24 hours after surgery. A large amount of bleeding is to be reported immediately. Concealed bleeding sometimes occurs in the wound, beneath the skin. If the clot formed is small, it will be absorbed by the body, but if large, the wound bulges and the clot must be removed for healing to continue.
- Infection: the second most frequent nosocomial (hospital acquired) infection in hospitals is surgical wound infections with Staphylococcus aureus, Escherichia coli, and Pseudomonas aeruginosa. Prevention is accomplished with meticulous wound management. Cellulitis is a bacterial infection that spreads into tissue planes. Systemic antibiotics are commonly prescribed. If the infection is in an arm or leg,

elevation of the limb reduces dependent edema and heat application promotes blood circulation. Abscess is a bacterial infection that is localized and characterized by pus. Treatment comprises of surgical drainage or excision with the concurrent administration of antibiotics.

- Dehiscence and evisceration: this condition results from sutures giving way, infection, distention, or cough. Pain results and the surgeon is called immediately. Prophylactically, an abdominal binder may be utilized.
- Keloid: refers to excessive growth of scar tissue. Careful wound closure, haemostasis, and pressure support are used to ward off this complication.

SURGICAL ASEPSIS

Aseptic technique is a set of specific practices and procedures performed under carefully controlled conditions with the goal of minimizing contamination by pathogens. Aseptic technique is employed to maximize and maintain asepsis, the absence of pathogenic organisms in the clinical setting. The goal of aseptic technique is to protect the patient from infection.

All patients are potentially vulnerable to infection. Certain situations further increase vulnerability, such as disturbance of the body's natural defences, such as occurs with extensive burns or an immune disorder. Typical situations that call for aseptic measures include surgery and the insertion of intravenous lines, urinary catheters, and drains.

The notion of asepsis can be applied in any clinical setting. Pathogens may introduce infection to the patient through contact with the environment, personnel, or equipment. The environment contains potential hazards that may spread pathogens through movement, touch, or proximity. Interventions such as controlling air flow by restricting traffic in the operating room, isolating a patient to protect airborne contamination, or using low-particle generating garb help to minimize environmental hazards.

A second element requiring careful attention is equipment or supplies. Medical equipment can be sterilized by chemical treatment, radiation, gas, or heat. Personnel can take steps to ensure sterility by evaluating that sterile packages are dry and intact and checking sterility indicators such as dates or coloured tape that changes colour when sterile.

Besides overall attention to the clinical environment and equipment, clinicians need to be attentive to their own practices and those of their peers in order to avoid inadvertent contamination.

A key difference between the operating room and other clinical environments is that the operating area has high standards of sterility at all times, while most other settings are not designed to meet such standards. However, the principles of aseptic technique can be applied in other clinical settings. The application of aseptic technique in such settings is termed "medical asepsis" or "clean technique" rather than "surgical asepsis" or "sterile technique" needed in the operating room.

Aseptic technique is most strictly applied in the operating room because of the direct and often extensive disruption of skin and underlying tissue. Aseptic technique helps to prevent or minimize postoperative infection. The patient is prepared or prepped by shaving hair from the surgical site, cleansing with a disinfectant such as iodine, and applying sterile drapes.

In all clinical settings, hand washing is a significant step in asepsis. In general settings, hands are to be washed when visibly soiled, before and after contact with the patient, after contact with other potential sources of micro-organisms, before invasive procedures, and after removal of gloves. Patients and visitors should also be encouraged to wash their hands. Proper hand washing for most clinical settings involves removal of jewellery, avoidance of clothing contact with the sink, and a minimum of 10-15 seconds scrubbing hands with soap, warm water, and vigorous friction.

A surgical scrub requires use of a long-acting, powerful, antimicrobial soap, careful scrubbing of the fingernails, and a longer period of time for scrubbing. Institutional policy commonly designates an acceptable minimum length of time needed. Thorough drying is essential, as moist surfaces invite the presence of pathogens. Contact after hand washing with the faucet or other potential contaminants should be avoided. The faucet can be turned off with a dry paper towel, or, in many cases, through use of foot pedals. Despite this careful scrub, bare hands are always considered potential sources of infection. A significant principle of aseptic technique is that fluid (a potential mode of pathogen transmission) flows in the direction of gravity. With this in mind, hands are held below elbows during the surgical scrub and above elbows following the surgical scrub.

Sterile surgical clothing or protective devices such as gloves, face masks, goggles, and transparent eye/face shields serve as a barrier against micro-organisms and are donned to maintain asepsis in the operating room. This practice includes covering facial hair, tucking hair out of sight, and removing jewellery or other dangling objects that may harbour unwanted organisms. This garb must be donned with deliberate care to avoid touching external, sterile surfaces with nonsterile objects including the skin. This ensures that potentially contaminated items such as hands and clothing remain behind protective barriers, thus prohibiting inadvertent entry of micro-organisms into sterile areas. Personnel assist the surgeon to don gloves and garb and arrange equipment to minimize the risk of contamination.

Donning sterile gloves requires specific technique so that the outer glove is not touched by the hand. A large cuff exposing the inner glove is created so that the glove may be grasped during donning. It is essential to avoid touching nonsterile items once sterile gloves are applied; the hands may be kept interlaced to avoid inadvertent contamination. Any break in the glove or touching the glove to a nonsterile surface requires immediate removal and application of new gloves.

Asepsis in the operating room or for other invasive procedures is also maintained by creating sterile surgical fields with drapes. Sterile drapes are sterilized linens placed on the patient or around the field to delineate sterile areas. Drapes or wrapped kits of equipment are opened in such a way that the contents do not touch non-sterile items or surfaces. Aspects of this method include opening the furthest areas of a package first, avoiding leaning over the contents, and preventing opened flaps from falling back onto contents.

CARE OF THE WOUND

A wound is a disruption in the continuity of cells-anything that causes cells that would typically be connected to become separated. Wound healing is the restoration of that continuity. Several effects may result with the occurrence of a wound: immediate loss of all or part of organ functioning, sympathetic stress response, haemorrhage and blood clotting, bacterial contamination, and death of cells. The most significant factor in minimizing these effects and promoting successful care is careful asepsis.

A biological process, wound healing begins with trauma and ends with scar formation. There are two types of tissue injury: full and partial thickness. Partial thickness injury is limited to the epidermis and superficial dermis with no damage to the dermal blood vessels. Healing occurs by regeneration of epithelial tissue. Full thickness injury involves loss of the dermis and extends to deeper tissue layers and disrupts dermal blood vessels. Wound healing involves the synthesis of several types of tissue and scar formation.

THREE PHASES OF REPAIR

The three phases of repair are "lag", "proliferative", and "remodelling". Directly after injury, haemostasis is achieved with clot formation. The fibrin clot acts like a highway for the migration of cells into the wound site. Within the first four hours of injury, neutrophils begin to appear. These inflammatory cells kill microbes, and prevent the colonization of the wound. Next the monocyte, or macrophage, appears. Functions of these cells include the killing of microbes, the breakdown of wound debris, and the secretion of cytokines that initiate the proliferative phase of repair. Synthetic cells, or fibroblasts, proliferate and synthesize new connective tissue, replacing the transitional fibrin matrix. At this time, an efficient nutrient supply develops through the arborization (terminal branching) of adjacent blood vessels. This ingrowth of new blood vessels is called angiogenesis. This new very vascularized connective tissue is referred to as granulation tissue.

Lag (inflammatory) phase: The first phase of repair is called the lag or inflammatory phase. The inflammatory response is dependent upon the depth and volume of tissue loss from the injury. Characteristics of the lag phase include acute inflammation and the initial appearance and infiltration of neutrophils. Neutrophils protect the host from micro-organisms and infection. If inflammation is delayed or stopped, the wound becomes susceptible to infection and closure is delayed.

Proliferative phase: The proliferative phase is the second phase of repair and is anabolic in nature. The lag and remodeling phase are both catabolic processes. The proliferative phase generates granulation tissue. In this process, acute inflammation releases cytokines, promoting fibroblast infiltration of the wound site, then creating a high density of cells. Collagen is the major connective tissue protein produced and released by fibroblasts. The connective tissue physically supports the new blood vessels that form and endothelial cells promote ingrowth of new vessels. These new blood vessels are necessary to meet the nutritional needs of the wound healing process.

Remodelling (maturation) phase: The mark of wound closure is when a new epidermal cover seals the defect. The process of wound healing continues underneath the new surface. This is the remodeling or maturation phase and is the third phase in healing.

THREE PRINCIPLES OF WOUND CARE

The first principle of wound care is the removal of non-viable tissue including necrotic (dead) tissue, slough, foreign debris, and residual material from dressings. Removal of non-viable tissue is referred to as debridement; removal of foreign matter is referred to as cleansing. Chronic wounds are colonized with bacteria, but not necessarily infected. A wound is colonized when a limited number of bacteria are present in the wound and are of no consequence in the healing process. A wound is infected when the bacterial burden overwhelms the immune response of the host and bacteria grow unchecked. Clinical signs of infection are redness of the skin around the wound, purulent (pus-containing) drainage, foul odour, and edema.

The second principle is providing a moist environment. This has been shown to promote re-epitheliazation and healing. Exposing wounds to air dries the surface and may impede the healing process. Gauze dressings provide a moist environment as long as they are kept moist in the wound. These are referred to as wet to dry dressings. Generally a saline soaked gauze dressing is loosely placed into the wound and covered with a dry gauze dressing to prevent drying and contamination. It also supports autolytic debridement (the body's own capacity to lyse and dissolve necrotic tissue), absorbs exudate, and traps bacteria in the gauze, which are removed when the dressing is changed.

Preventing further injury is the third principle of wound care. This involves elimination or reduction of the condition that allowed the wound to develop. Factors that contribute to the development of chronic wounds include losses in mobility, mental status changes, deficits of sensation, and circulatory deficits. Patients must be correctly positioned to eradicate continued pressure to the chronic wound. Pressure reducing devices, such as mattresses, cushions, supportive boots, foam wedges, and fitted shoes can be used to keep pressure off wounds.

Providing nutrition, specifically protein for healing, is the fourth principle of healing. Protein is essential for wound repair and regeneration. Without essential amino acids, angiogenesis, fibroblast proliferation, collagen synthesis, and scar remodelling will not occur. Amino acids also support the immune response. Adequate amounts of carbohydrates and fats are required to prevent the amino acids from being oxidized for caloric needs. Glucose is also required to meet the energy requirements of the cells involved in wound repair. Albumin is the most significant indicator of malnutrition because it is sacrificed to provide essential amino acids if there is inadequate protein intake.

COMPONENTS OF WOUND CARE

Effective wound care begins with an evaluation of the entire patient. This includes obtaining a complete health history and a physical evaluation.

Evaluating the patient assists in identifying causes and contributing factors of the wound. When examining the wound, it is significant to document its size, location, appearance, and the surrounding skin. The health care professional also examines the wound for exudate, necrotic tissue, signs of infection, and drainage, and documents how long the patient has had the wound. It is also significant to know what treatment, if any, the patient has previously received for the wound.

Actual components of wound care include cleaning, dressing, determining frequency of dressing changes, and reeavaluation. Removing dead tissue and debris that impedes healing, is the goal of cleaning the wound. When cleaning the wound, protective goggles should be worn and sterile saline solution should be used. Providone iodine, sodium hypochlorite, and hydrogen peroxide should never be used, as they are toxic to cells.

Cleaning

Gentle pressure should be used to clean the wound if there is no necrotic tissue. This can be accomplished by utilizing a 60 cc catheter tip syringe to apply the cleaning solution. If the wound has necrotic tissue, more pressure may be required. Whirlpools can also be used for wounds having a thick layer of exudate. At times, chemical or surgical debridement may be required to remove debris.

Dressing

Dressings are applied to wounds for the following reasons: to provide the proper environment for healing, to absorb drainage, to immobilize the wound, to protect the wound and new tissue growth from mechanical injury and bacterial contamination, to promote haemostasis, and to provide mental/physical patient comfort. Bandages and dressings are both used in wound management. A bandage is a piece of cloth or other material used to bind or wrap a diseased or injured part of the body. Commonly shaped as a strip or pad, bandages are either placed directly against the wound or used to bind a dressing to the wound. A dressing can consist of a wide range of materials, sometimes containing medication, placed against the wound.

The intentions served by dressings include protecting wounds; promoting healing; and providing, retaining, or removing moisture. Bandages can be used to hold dressings in place, and also to relieve pain and generally make the patient comfortable. Elastic bandages are useful to provide ongoing pressure on varicose veins, fractured ribs, swollen joints, etc.

There have been tremendous advances made in the design and composition of dressings and bandages in recent years. The field is becoming increasingly complex, and there are numerous reports of health care workers applying inappropriate products.

REFERENCES

Allen, J. B. (1998). An acupuncture treatment study for unipolar depression. Psychological Science, 9, 397–401.

Astin, J. A. (1998). Why patients use alternative medicine: Results of a national study. Journal of American Medical Association, 279(19), 1548–1553.

Benson, H. (1975). The relaxation response. New York: William Morrow.

Bowlby, J. (1984). Attachment and loss: Volume 1: Attachment (2nd ed.). London: Penguin Books.

Brinker, F. (1997). Herbal contraindications and drug interactions. Sandy, OR: Eclectic Institute.

Buckle, J. (1997). Clinical aromatherapy in nursing. London: Hodder Headline Group.

Burmeister, A. (1997). The touch of healing: Energizing body, mind, and spirit with Jin Shu Jyutsu. New York: Bantam Books.

Campbell, J. (1998). The riddle of the Mozart effect. Natural Health, (Jan-Feb), 114–119.

Cardini, F., & Weixin, H. (1998). Moxibustion for correction of breech presentation: A randomized controlled trial. Journal of the American Medical Association, 280, 1580–1584.

13

Special Needs of the Patient

HYPERTHERMIA/HYPOTHERMIA MANAGEMENT

Hyperthermia/hypothermia unit management is the use of special electronically regulated blankets or pads to adjust body temperature until it returns to normal levels. The human body operates at temperatures within a fairly narrow range.

A body temperature of 98.6°F (Fahrenheit), or 37°C (Celsius), is considered to be normal for human beings. In reality, normal body temperature varies not only in different individuals, but also in the same person, depending upon activities engaged in or the time of day. Exercise, eating, and ovulation in women can raise body temperature, while sleeping, drinking fluids, and (for women) menses can lower it. Body temperature is typically at its lowest level at 3 A.M. and at its highest level at 6 P.M. However, all of these variations do not normally extend beyond a range of 97.8°F (36.5°C) and 99°F (37.2°C).

The purpose of hyperthermia and hypothermia units is to correct aberrant temperature and prevent the complications that can occur when this narrow range of human body temperature is not maintained. Sometimes, body temperature is purposefully lowered to aid in certain surgical procedures. The lower body temperature allows vital organs such as the heart to survive with decreased blood supply, thus increasing the available time a surgeon has to operate. But the usual reason hyperthermia or hypothermia equipment is used is because the body has exceeded the extremes in temperature. Normally, a section of the brain known as the hypothalamus acts to regulate temperature in a manner similar to the workings of a thermostat.

Body temperature is constantly monitored by the hypothalamus, and mechanisms to compensate for any abnormality are set in motion. Classic examples of such mechanisms are shivering and perspiring. The hypothalamus reacts to low body temperature by sending neurological impulses that cause shivering. Shivering in turn produces heat from within the body through muscle activity. When the body temperature rises, the hypothalamus causes fluid to be excreted via the skin as perspiration. As the perspiration evaporates, it lowers the body temperature. Both excessively high and low temperatures can be medical emergencies capable of causing death without immediate, appropriate medical intervention.

Among the causes of abnormally elevated or lowered temperature are:

- Exposure to extreme heat or cold
- Infections
- Glandular disorders, especially those that involve the thyroid gland
- Certain tumours
- Abnormal reaction to anaesthesia
- Dehydration

Usually, hyperthermia is a pathological condition. Patients whose temperature rises above 105.8°F (41°C) are considered to be at serious risk of brain damage, and those with a temperature above 109.4°F (43° C) will usually not survive. Mental confusion and delirium seizures (especially in young children and infants) are some of the serious problems associated with high fevers. Hypothermia is medically defined as a drop in body temperature to below 95°F (35°C). Hypothermia can lead to irregular heartbeat and, eventually, cardiac arrest. The elderly and very young children are the most vulnerable to extreme drops in body temperature. The Merck Manual recommends that health care staff consider people with radically low body temperature as viable and treatable until the body has been warmed, and there are still no signs of life such as heartbeat and respirations. Length of exposure to cold and general health are standard predictors of survival, but the National Institute on Aging gives the following guidelines regarding the chances of recovery for hypothermia victims:

- If body temperature has not fallen below 90°F (32.2°C), the likelihood of complete recovery is good.
- When body temperature is between 80°F (26.6°C) and 90°F (32,2°C), the majority of hypothermia victims survive, but are likely to have lasting damage such as brain damage.

- People with temperatures below 80°F (26.6°C) are not likely to live.

Hypothermia/hyperthermia units should never be placed in direct contact with the patient's skin due to the risk of burns. For centuries, wrapping feverish people in cold, wet sheets and immersing them in cool baths helped to lower body temperature. Hot water bottles and blankets were used to warm hypothermia victims. Today, hyperthermia blankets or pads are special medical devices that have a built-in temperature regulator, or thermostat, capable of raising or lowering body temperature. Such blankets or pads circulate solution through them at pre-set temperature levels calculated to raise or lower body temperature.

There are various kinds, and manufacturer's instructions for each type must be read and understood. Some utilize dry cold to lower temperature, and are used for just one patient and then discarded. Others have a special adapter to change from heat to cold, and can be used again and again. A K-Pad is one brand of pad used in some health care facilities to raise the temperature in hypothermia victims. K-Pads are composed of tubular forms that are filled with water, which is then heated and monitored by an electronic thermostat to keep it at the correct temperature.

PREPARATION OF PATIENT

Often, the patient with a radical alteration in temperature may be unconscious. But if the person is aware, providing a good explanation of what is being done and why will be very important. Although some brands of hyperthermia/hypothermia blankets are cloth-covered, patients should still always have a bath blanket beneath and over them so that their skin does not come in direct contact with the hyperthermia/hypothermia equipment.

This is particularly important when the unit is being used to warm the body, as direct contact can result in burns. KPads are filled two-thirds full of water, and superfluous air is removed before use. Most hyperthermia/hypothermia units have dual temperature monitors for both the temperature of the unit and that of the patient. This temperature probe for the person often involves a rectal probe, as that is the most accurate measure of body temperature.

Regardless, it is imperative that the person's temperature be monitored constantly, and if the unit does not measure body temperature, then the temperature must be taken with a regular thermometer. (In the case of hypothermia, a special thermometer that registers below 94°F [34.4°C] will be necessary.)

AFTERCARE

In the case of hyperthermia, the cooling unit is removed while the body temperature is still slightly above normal, as the body will continue to cool after the unit is removed. The temperature continues to be monitored, and cold packs to axillae (the armpits) and the groins may also be used. Often, fever-reducing medications such as acetaminophen are given once the person is conscious, or may be administered by suppository. The vital signs (temperature, pulse, respirations, and blood pressure) continue to be monitored for hypothermia patients. The warming unit is not usually removed until the body temperature rises to normal. Warm liquids may be given once the person is conscious.

COMPLICATIONS

The major complication involved in the use of hypothermia/ hyperthermia units is either the occurrence of burns from units used for heating or the discomfort from more direct contact with cooling units. Both can be prevented by following procedures, including the placement of bath blankets between the patient and the unit and reading the manufacturer's instructions. Optimum results from the use of these units are a return to normal bodily temperature without the person sustaining any permanent damage.

HEALTH CARE TEAM ROLES

Emergency personnel such as emergency room technicians (EMTs) and physicians are often involved as both hypothermia and hyperthermia are often accidental happenings, occurring due to exposure to heat or cold sustained from immersion in water or being exposed to the elements. Also, registered nurses (RNs) and licensed practical nurses (LPNs) are responsible for setting up hypothermia/ hyperthermia units and caring for the patient undergoing temperature-altering treatment.

SENSORIUM

Nursing the unconscious patient can be a challenging experience. Unconscious patients have no control over themselves or their environment and thus are highly dependent on the nurse. The skills needed to care for unconscious patients are not specific to critical care and theatres as unconscious patients are nursed in a variety of clinical settings. Nursing such patients can be a source of anxiety for nurses. However, with a good knowledge base to initiate the evaluation, planning and implementation of quality care, nursing patients who are unconscious can prove highly rewarding, and the skills acquired can promote confidence in the care of all patients. Unconsciousness spans a broad spectrum, from momentary loss of consciousness as seen with fainting, to prolonged coma that may last weeks, months or even years. The causes of unconsciousness will dictate the length of the coma and the prognosis. Yet the immediate and ongoing needs of the unconscious patient are similar, whatever the underlying cause.

To understand consciousness it is necessary to have an appreciation of the complexity of the related anatomy and physiology, as normal conscious behaviour is dependent on an intact and fully functioning brain. Therefore, the manifestation of impaired or absent consciousness points towards an underlying brain dysfunction.

Consciousness can be defined as a state of awareness of one's self and the environment. A conscious individual is capable of responding to sensory stimuli. Alternatively, coma is a total absence of awareness of one's self and the environment. An individual in a coma is unrousable and unresponsive to external stimuli. For instance, when an individual is asleep he or she can be aroused by external stimuli, but this does not occur when an individual is in a coma. This suggests that consciousness depends on whether the individual can be aroused to wakefulness. However, between the poles of consciousness and unconsciousness there is a continuum of differing states of impaired consciousness.

URINARY ELIMINATION

Urinary incontinence (UI) is a multifactorial syndrome produced by a combination of genitourinary pathology, age-related changes, and comorbid conditions that impair normal micturition or the functional ability to toilet oneself, or both. The prevalence of UI increases with age and affects women more than men (2: 1) until age 80, after which men and women are evenly affected. Of persons aged 65 years and over, 15% to 30% in the community and at least 50% in long-term care are incontinent. UI can cause morbidity, including cellulitis, pressure ulcers, urinary tract infections, falls with fractures, sleep deprivation, social withdrawal, depression, and sexual dysfunction. UI is not associated with increased mortality. UI impairs quality of life, affecting the older person's emotional well-being, social function, and general health. Incontinent persons often manage to maintain their activities, but with an increased burden of coping, embarrassment, and poor self-perception. Caregiver burden is higher with incontinent older persons, which can contribute to decisions to hospitalize. Estimated annual UI-related costs total more than $36 billion.

For older persons in particular, continence requires mobility, manual dexterity, the cognitive ability to recognize and react to bladder filling, and the motivation to stay dry. Bladder smooth muscle (the detrusor) contracts via parasympathetic nerves from spinal cord levels S2 to S4. Urethral sphincter mechanisms include proximal urethral smooth muscle (which contracts with sympathetic stimulation from spinal levels T11 to L2), distal urethral striated muscle (which contracts via cholinergic somatic stimulation from cord levels S2 to S4), and musculofascial urethral supports. In women, these supports form a two-layered "hammock" that supports and compresses the urethra when abdominal pressure increases. Micturition is coordinated by the central nervous system: Parietal lobes and thalamus receive and coordinate detrusor afferent stimuli; frontal lobes and basal ganglia provide signals to inhibit voiding; and the pontine micturition centre integrates these inputs into socially appropriate voiding with coordinated urethral relaxation and detrusor contraction until the bladder is empty. Urine storage is under sympathetic control (inhibiting detrusor contraction and increasing sphincter tone), and voiding is parasympathetic (detrusor contractor and relaxation of sphincter tone).

ASSESSMENT

The multifactorial nature of UI in older persons requires a comprehensive diagnostic assessment, with a careful search for all possible causes and precipitants beyond a focus on specific genitourinary diagnoses.

Routine urodynamic testing is optional and commonly is not required. Precise diagnosis is most significant when surgical treatment is being considered for stress UI or outlet obstruction, because surgery is ineffective for DO, DHIC, and detrusor weakness that present with similar symptoms. Geriatric UI is multifactorial, and lower urinary tract pathology is rarely the only cause. A focus on urodynamic diagnosis detracts from more relevant precipitants. Moreover, some treatments are effective for several types of UI. Thus, urodynamics should be considered only before surgical intervention, if the diagnosis is unclear, or when empiric therapy has failed. Cystometry determines only bladder proprioception, capacity, detrusor stability, and contractility; carbon dioxide cystometry may be unreliable. Simultaneous measurement of abdominal pressure is necessary to exclude abdominal straining and detect DHIC. Fluoroscopic monitoring, abdominal leak-point pressure, or profilometry tests detect and quantify stress UI. Pressure-flow studies detect obstruction. Peak urine flow rates 12 mL per second (without straining for voids of at least 150 to 200 mL) reliably exclude obstruction. Low flow rates are nondiagnostic, and precise diagnosis requires urodynamic assessment.

Bedside cystometry may detect DO and measure bladder capacity. The PVR is measured by catheterization; then the bladder is filled through a syringe attached to the catheter. DO is identified by a rise in fluid level in the syringe column. Though bedside cystometry has moderate sensitivity and specificity for DO in ambulatory older persons, its true utility is unclear. Among community-dwelling older persons, its benefit over history and physical examination is unknown. When it is used in long-term-care patients, low-pressure DHIC contractions can be missed, and it may be difficult to differentiate DO from abdominal straining.

MANAGEMENT

Because age-related changes render older persons more vulnerable to developing UI from factors such as medical illnesses and medications, correction of those factors alone often improves continence. Relieving the most bothersome aspects of UI for the patient is key. A stepped strategy moving from least to more invasive treatments should be used, with behavioural methods tried before medication, and both tried before surgery. Treatment that simply decreases the number of UI episodes may not be sufficient for persons most bothered by the timing of UI, nocturia, or leakage with exercise.

FUNCTIONING OF SENSORY ORGANS: (VISUAL & HEARING IMPAIRMENT)

Patients who are hearing impaired or deaf are commonly not ashamed or embarrassed by their disability. Often, it is the people around a deaf or hearing-impaired individual who have the problem coping. Remember that you must be able to communicate with hearing-impaired patients so that you can provide necessary or even lifesaving care.

The vast majority of hearing-impaired patients have normal intelligence. Hearing-impaired patients can commonly understand what is going on around them, provided that you can successfully communicate with them. Most patients who are hearing impaired can read lips to some extent. Therefore, the nurse should place herself in a position so that the patient can see her lips. Many hearing-impaired patients have hearing aids to help them communicate. Be careful that hearing aids are not lost during an accident or fall. Not only are they extremely expensive, hearing aids will often make it easier to communicate. Hearing aids may also be forgotten if the patient is confused or ill.

Like hearing-impaired patients, visually impaired and blind patients have commonly accepted and learned to deal with their disability. Of course, not all visually impaired patients are completely blind. Many can perceive light and dark or can see shadows or movement. The nurse should ask the patient whether he or she can see at all. The nurse should also remember that as with other patients who have disability, she should expect that visually impaired patients have normal intelligence. As she begin caring for a visually impaired patient, explain everything in detail that what she is doing. She should stay in physical contact with the patient as she begin their care. She should avoid sudden movements. She should ensure that if the patient can walk to the ambulance, place his or her hand on her own arm, taking care not to rush. Transport any mobility aids, such as a cane, with the patient to the hospital. A visually impaired individual may have a guide dog. Guide dogs are easily identified by their special harness. They are trained not to leave their masters and not to respond to strangers.

ASSESSMENT OF SELF CARE ABILITY

In the evaluation of self care ability a nurse should perform following activities:

- Recognize that a person's bodymind- spirit has healing capacities that can be developed and supported through self-care practices.
- Identify and integrate self-care strategies to develop their physical, psychological, sociological, and spiritual well-being.
- Recognize and address at-risk health patterns and begin the process of change.
- Consciously cultivate awareness and understanding about the deeper meaning, intention, inner strengths, and connections with self, others, nature, and God/Life Force/Absolute/ Transcendent.
- Use clear intention to care for self and to seek a sense of balance, harmony, and joy in daily life.
- Participate in the evolutionary holistic process with the understanding that crisis creates opportunity in any setting.

COMMUNICATION METHODS AND SPECIAL CONSIDERATION

The Nurse should always remember that evaluation of the activity of communicating is only part of a holistic nursing evaluation and should not be undertaken in isolation without reference to or consideration of the client's other activities of living. The specific points to consider when evaluating a client's ability to communicate include:

PHYSICAL

- Are their senses intact?
- Do they have any disorder or diseases affecting their sensory organs, for instance laryngeal palsy, tinnitus, cerebral vascular accident (CVA)?
- Are they able to hear satisfactorily?
- Do they require any hearing aids? Are these functioning?
- How does the individual typically communicate: do they lip read, sign or
- Braille or use any speech aids such as a possum, robot or speaking tube?
- Do they have any speech impediment or impairment?
- Are they able to gesticulate, show affection or distaste?
- Can they control pitch and/or tone?
- Can they see satisfactorily or do they have/need spectacles or contact lenses?
- Can they read and/or write?
- Is their cognitive ability impaired?
- Are there any physiological signs of nervousness, for instance dilated pupils, tremor, perspiration?

PSYCHOLOGICAL

- Are they worried, nervous or frightened?
- Are they depressed, anxious or excitable?
- What is their level of intelligence?
- Can they understand complex language?
- What is their range of vocabulary?
- Are they self-confident/timid?
- Do they seem angry or upset? Are there any signs of actual or potential aggression or violence?

SOCIOCULTURAL

- What is their first language or mother tongue?

- Do they possess a second or third language and if so how fluent are they?
- Do they understand the local dialect and colloquialisms?
- Are there any cultural issues surrounding communication and body language, for instance social status, eye contact, proximity or touch?
- Do they use any unfamiliar jargon or abbreviations?
- Do they need an interpreter?

ENVIRONMENTAL

- Is the environment too hot, too cold or poorly ventilated?
- Is it too light or too dark?
- Does the client prefer a quiet environment or do they prefer background noise?
- Do they wish to communicate in a more private place or are they happy to discuss issues at the bedside in hearing distance of others?
- Are there any physical barriers to communication, for instance furniture arrangement, size or type of room?
- Is the environment safe for client, self and others should the client become aggressive or violent?

POLITICO-ECONOMIC

- What communication channels does the individual use or prefer, for instance telephone, newspapers, TV, email, Internet?
- Is the individual computer literate?
- Are they familiar with their rights/duties, for instance Data Protection Act?

Some of the barriers to effective communication are listed below:

- Failing to undertake a holistic evaluation
- Failing to establish or explain the intention of the interaction
- Failing to listen
- Failure to establish an environment of warmth and acceptance
- Personality, for instance an individual who is shy or introverted or, conversely, one who is domineering
- Lack of trust

- False reassurance
- Physical state, for instance too tired or in too much pain
- Layout of furniture, for instance sitting behind a desk or table
- Emotional state, for instance too angry to listen
- Stress; seeming to be too busy
- Lack of privacy
- Visual impairment
- Environmental noise
- Hearing impairment
- Preoccupied
- Personal attitudes and values
- Status
- Religious/cultural beliefs
- Culture of the ward/institution
- Using closed questions inappropriately
- Using inappropriate language, colloquialisms and jargon
- Using leading questions inappropriately
- Misinterpreting or failing to clarify the essence of what has been or is being said
- Inappropriate use of facts
- Interrupting

PAIN

Pain is a universal human experience; it is defined as "a state in which an individual experiences and reports the presence of severe discomfort or an uncomfortable sensation". Pain is a subjective experience that is often difficult for clients to describe and nurses to understand, yet it is among the most common complaints that cause individuals to seek health care. McCaffery and Pasero (1999) recognize the subjective nature of pain by stating "Pain is whatever the experiencing person says it is, existing whenever he says it does". Until recently, pain was viewed as a symptom that required diagnosis and treatment of the underlying cause. It is now clear that pain itself can be detrimental to the health and healing of clients. "Unrelieved pain is not only detrimental, it's avoidable". Pain is a stressor that can trigger both physiological and psychological discomfort.

Untreated pain can lead to physical disorders related to undernutrition, immobility, and immune suppression.

NATURE OF PAIN

Pain, a response to noxious stimuli, can be a protective mechanism to prevent further injury, as is seen in clients who guard or protect an injured body part. The sensation of pain as the warning of potential tissue damage may be absent in people with nerve/spinal cord abnormalities, diabetic neuropathy, multiple sclerosis, and nerve/spinal cord injury.

TYPES OF PAIN

Pain can be qualified or described in two basic ways: By its cause or origin and by its description or nature.

Pain categorized by its origin is either cutaneous, somatic, or visceral. Cutaneous pain is caused by stimulation of the cutaneous nerve endings in the skin and results in a well-localized "burning" or "prickling" sensation; getting a knot in the hair that is pulled out during combing may cause cutaneous pain. Somatic pain is nonlocalized and originates in support structures such as tendons, ligaments, and nerves; jamming a knee or finger will result in somatic pain. Visceral pain is discomfort in the internal organs and is less localized and more slowly transmitted than cutaneous pain. Visceral pain is often difficult to assess because the location may not be directly related to the cause. Pain originating from the abdominal organs is often called referred pain because the sensation of pain is not felt in the organ itself but instead is perceived at the spot where the organs were located during foetal development.

Acute pain is most frequently identified by its sudden onset and relatively short duration, mild to severe intensity, and a steady decrease in intensity over a period of days to weeks. Some forms of acute pain may have a slower onset. Once the noxious stimulus is resolved, the pain usually decreases. Examples of noxious stimuli are needle sticks, surgical incisions, burns, and fractures.

Recurrent acute pain is identified by repetitive painful episodes that may recur over a prolonged period or throughout the client's lifetime. These painful episodes alternate with pain-free intervals. Examples of recurrent pain include migraine headaches, sickle cell pain crises, and the pain of angina pectoris due to myocardial hypoxia.

Chronic pain is identified as long-term (lasting 6 months or longer), persistent, nearly constant, or recurrent pain that produces significant negative changes in the client's life. Unlike acute pain, chronic pain may last long after the pathology is resolved.

Chronic acute pain occurs almost daily over a long period, has the potential for lasting months or years, and has a high probability of ending. Severe burn injuries and cancer are examples of pathophysiology that leads to chronic acute pain, which may last for long periods before the condition is cured or controlled.

Chronic nonmalignant pain (CNP), occurs almost daily and lasts for at least 6 months, with intensity ranging from mild to severe. Chronic pain, a primary motivator for individuals to seek health care intervention, can greatly influence a client's quality of life, including emotional, social, vocational, and financial areas. There is a relationship between chronic conditions (including pain) and depression. Thus, the client experiencing chronic pain should always be assessed for the presence of depression. "Not only do patients with CNP have a higher rate of depression, but suicide potential is also a serious concern for this population". Examples of pathophysiology leading to chronic nonmalignant pain include:

- Many forms of neuralgia (paroxysmal pain that extends along the course of one or more nerves)
- Low back pain
- Rheumatoid arthritis
- Ankylosing spondylitis
- Phantom limb pain (a form of neuropathic pain that occurs after amputation with pain sensations referred to an area in the missing portion of the limb)
- Myofascial pain syndromes (a group of muscle disorders characterized by pain, muscle spasm, tenderness, stiffness, and limited motion) CNP may be associated with several problems, including:
- Activity intolerance, which leads to physical deconditioning
- Functional impairment with resultant changes in role performance (parent, breadwinner) o Social isolation, which alters relationships
- Sleep deprivation
- Frustration, anxiety, anger, and depression When CNP is severe enough to disable the client, nurses understand that in order "To improve your patient's quality of life, pain management becomes a priority".

FACTORS AFFECTING THE PAIN

The subjective nature of pain varies from person to person and is influenced by several variables. Many factors account for the differences in a client's individual response to pain, including age, previous experience with pain, and cultural factors.

Age

Age can greatly influence a client's perception of the pain experience. Infants are sensitive to pain and typically exhibit discomfort through crying or physical movement. Toddlers also use crying and physical movement to indicate pain, and they begin to develop the skills needed to verbally describe pain or point to the area that is hurting. Children often do not understand why pain occurs and can therefore be frightened or resentful of the pain experience; in some cases, children revert to habits of their younger years (regression) as a coping mechanism when faced with pain they cannot otherwise manage. Adolescents often sense great peer pressure and may be reluctant to admit having pain for fear of being called weak or sensitive.

Adults may continue pain behaviours they learned as children and may also be reluctant to admit pain or seek medical care because of fear of the unknown or fear of the impact that treatment may have on their lifestyle. Older adults may often ignore their pain, viewing it as an unavoidable consequence of aging; family and health care members may inadvertently support this stereotype and be less than responsive to an older client's complaints of pain. Pain related to chronic disease is prevalent among the elderly population. Up to 70% of noninstutionalized older adults report the occurrence of pain. Frequently, pain is undertreated in older people. Loeb (1999) states that there are three major factors which contribute to inadequate pain management in older clients:

- Pain is underreported by older people who believe the myth that pain is a normal part of aging. Older adults with such misconceptions believe nothing can be done to relieve the pain.
- Underdetection of pain may be a result of the client's cognitive-perceptual deficits.
- Undertreatment of pain is a result of underreporting and underdetection.

Previous Experience

Clients' previous exposures to pain will often influence their reactions. Coping mechanisms that were used in the past may affect clients' judgments as to how the pain will affect their lives and what measures they can use to successfully manage the pain on their own. Client teaching about pain expectations and management methods can often allay client fears and lead to more successful pain management, especially in those clients who do not have previous pain experience or who have memories of a previous devastating pain experience that they do not wish to repeat.

Cultural Norms

Cultural diversity in pain responses can easily lead to problems in pain management. There are no significant differences among groups in the level of intensity at which pain becomes appreciable or perceptible. However, the level of intensity or duration of pain the client is willing to endure is culturally determined. Expression of pain is also governed by cultural values. In some cultures, tolerance to pain, and therefore "suffering in silence," is expected; in others, full expression of pain may include animated physical and emotional responses. The nurse must be careful not to equate the level of expression of pain with the level of actual pain experienced, but to instead consider cultural influences that affect the expression of pain.

NURSING ASSESSMENT

Assessment of pain includes collection of subjective and objective data through the use of various assessment tools and construction of a database to use in developing a pain management plan. Pain assessment should be performed for every client. In the normal course of doing business, pain should be nursing's fifth vital sign, as basic to practice as temperature, pulse, respiration, and blood pressure. Cheever emphasizes the need to prevent pain rather than treat it. Prevention calls for accurate assessment in order to alleviate pain before it escalates. Even if a patient fails to report pain, you must make efforts to detect it. Gathering subjective information regarding the client's pain is the first step in pain assessment.

The client's perception of the pain should cover a description of several qualifiers, including:

- Aggravating factors (variables that worsen the pain, such as exercise, certain foods, or stress)
- Alleviating factors (measures the client can take that lessen the effect of the pain, such as lying down, avoiding certain foods, or taking medication)
- Associated manifestations (factors that often accompany the pain, such as nausea, constipation, or dizziness)

- Intensity
- Location
- Quality (radiating, burning, diffuse)

Nurses must look for nonverbal signs of pain such as changes in motor activity or facial expression. It is also important to ask family members to share their observations; they may be the first ones to note subtle behaviour changes indicative of pain. When assessing a client's report of pain, the nurse should also determine a client's pain threshold and pain tolerance level. Pain threshold is the level of intensity at which pain becomes appreciable or perceptible and will vary with each individual and type of pain. Pain tolerance is the level of intensity or duration of pain the client is willing or able to endure. A client's perceptions and attitudes about pain are dramatically influenced by many factors, including previous experiences and cultural background. Clients' behavioural adaptation may yield no report of pain unless questioned specifically.

MANAGEMENT

Below are listed some recommendations on caring for clients experiencing pain.

- Recognize each client's right to pain assessment and treatment
- Monitor client responses to pain management strategies
- Educate staff and clients about pain management
- Clients have the right to appropriate pain assessment
- Pain is to be assessed and regularly reassessed.
- Clients will be treated for pain or referred for treatment.
- Clients will be taught the importance of effective pain management.
- Clients will be taught that pain management is a part of treatment.
- Clients will be involved in making health care decisions.
- Analgesics are to be administered as needed.
- Discharge planning and teaching will include continuing needs for pain management.

Establishment of a therapeutic relationship is the foundation for effective nursing care of the client experiencing pain. Clients who trust their nurses to be there, to listen, and to act, are the clients who are most likely to be comfortable. Client education regarding pain management begins with defining pain, identifying the probable causes, introducing clients to pain assessment tools, and allowing them to choose the tool they would like to use. The importance of talking with health care providers about their pain and of using a preventive approach to pain management must also be emphasized. Provide written information to reinforce verbal explanations.

Teach the importance of around-the-clock dosing instead of PRN administration of analgesic medications. Refer to the Client Teaching Checklist for pain management information. When a client is to be discharged from a health care facility, discharge teaching should include pain management information with specific guidelines about the need for seeking follow-up advice/treatment.

Both nonpharmacologic and pharmacologic interventions can be effective in caring for clients with pain. In some cases of mild pain, nonpharmacologic techniques may be the primary intervention, with medication available as "backup." In cases of moderate to severe pain, nonpharmacologic techniques can be an effective adjunctive, or complementary treatment.

Pharmacologic Pain Management

Listed below are principles for the care of clients experiencing pain:

- Assess the pain.
- Treat the contributing factors (pathology).
- Individualize analgesic therapy to each client.
- Choose the least invasive route of administration.
- Administer analgesics at regularly scheduled intervals (around-the-clock dosing) rather than on an as needed (PRN) basis.
- Keep clients in control of their own analgesia as much as possible.
- Titrate doses to provide maximum pain relief and minimum side effects. Know that the right dose is whatever it takes to relieve the pain with the fewest side effects.

TREATMENTS RELATED TO GASTROINTESTINAL SYSTEM

Nasogastric Suction

Nasogastric suction is the process of removing solids, liquids, or gasses from the stomach or small intestine by inserting a tube through the nose and suctioning the material through the tube. This procedure may be done in the following situations:

- To relieve pressure on the stomach or small intestine when intestinal obstruction is suspected.
- Before operations on the stomach or intestines.
- To obtain a sample of the stomach contents for analysis.
- To remove toxic substances.
- To flush the stomach during gastrointestinal bleeding or poisonings.

For this procedure, the patient sits upright while a lubricated tube is slipped through the nose and down the throat. The patient may be asked to sip water at a certain point in the procedure to help the tube slide in more easily. If the tube is to be placed into the small intestine, the doctor may use an endoscope (a thin, flexible instrument containing a camera and a light) to help see where the tube is going. Once the tube is in place, material can be removed from the stomach or intestines with gentle suction.

Different types of nasogastric tubes are used for different intentions. Tubes used for stomach flushing are called orogastric tubes and are the largest in diameter. Tubes that are threaded through the lower opening of the stomach (pylorus) and into the small intestine are stiffer and have a balloon tip.

Most patients tolerate nasogastric suctioning well. After the tube is removed, the patient's throat may feel irritated, but no special care is required. The most serious risk from this procedure is that the patient will inhale some of the stomach contents into the lungs (aspiration). This may lead to bronchial infections and aspiration pneumonia. There is also the chance that the tube will be misplaced in the windpipe (trachea), causing violent coughing. Irritation to the throat and esophagus can cause bleeding.

GASTRIC IRRIGATION

Gastritis usually refers to inflammation of the lining of the stomach, but the term is often used to cover a variety of symptoms resulting from stomach lining inflammation and symptoms of burning or discomfort. True gastritis comes in several forms and is diagnosed using a combination of tests. In the 1990s, scientists discovered that the main cause of true gastritis is infection from a bacterium called Helicobacter pylori (H. pylori).

Gastritis should not be confused with common symptoms of upper abdominal discomfort. It has been associated with resulting ulcers, particularly peptic ulcers. And in some cases, chronic gastritis can lead to more serious complications. The main cause of true gastritis is H. pylori infection. H. pylori is indicated in an average of 90% of patients with chronic gastritis.

A procedure used to empty the stomach of its contents. Performed using a flexible rubber tube that is passed through the mouth and advanced to the stomach. This procedure includes the instillation of a balanced salt solution into the stomach (via the tube) followed by suctioning the fluid out of the stomach. An effective procedure in the treatment of toxic ingestions.

Gastric lavage involves the passage of a tube via the mouth or nose down into the stomach, followed by sequential administration and removal of small volumes of liquid. The placement of the tube in the stomach must be confirmed either by air insufflation while listening to the stomach, by pH testing a small amount of aspirated stomach contents, or x-ray. This is to ensure the tube is not in the lungs. In adults, small amounts of warm water or saline are administered and via a siphoning action removed again. In children, normal saline is used, as children are more at risk of developing hyponatremia if lavaged with water. Because of the possibility of vomiting, a suction device is always on hand in case of pulmonary aspiration of stomach contents. Lavage is repeated until the returning fluid shows no further gastric contents. If the patient is unconscious or cannot protect their airway then the patient should be intubated before performing lavage.

GASTRIC ANALYSIS

Gastric analysis comprises of a series of tests used to analyze the contents of the stomach. The complete series involves:

- Collecting residual gastric fluid from a fasting patient
- Collecting basal secretions every 15 minutes for four hours
- Intramuscular administration of a drug that stimulates gastric acid output
- Collecting stomach secretions every 15 minutes for 90 minutes

The appearance, blood, bile, pH, volume, millimoles of H+ per liter, millimoles of H+ per volume, and millimoles of H+ per hour of each specimen is then evaluated. A gastric analysis is performed to evaluate gastric function by measuring the contents of a fasting patient's stomach the for acidity, appearance, and volume. The basal gastric secretion test is indicated for patients with obscure gastric pain, loss of appetite, and weight loss. It is also utilized for suspected peptic ulcer, severe gastritis, and Zollinger-Ellison (Z-E) syndrome.

The gastric acid stimulation test is indicated when abnormalities are found during the basal secretion test. These abnormalities can be caused by a number of disorders, including duodenal ulcer, pernicious anaemia, and gastric cancer. While this test will detect abnormalities, x rays and other studies are necessary to obtain a definitive diagnosis. Because both the basal acid output test and the gastric acid stimulation test require gastric intubation through the mouth or nasal passage, neither test is recommended for patients with oesophageal problems, aortic aneurysm, severe gastric haemorrhage, or congestive heart failure. The gastric acid output test is also not recommended in patients who are sensitive to pentagastrin (the drug used to stimulate gastric acid output).

This test, whether performed for basal gastric acid secretion, gastric acid stimulation, or both, requires gastric intubation by mouth or through the nasal passage. The patient should be fasting overnight (12 hours) prior to intubation. After allowing approximately 10 to 15 minutes for the patient to adjust to the presence of the tube, and with the patient in a sitting position, specimens are obtained every 15 minutes for a period of 90 minutes. The first two specimens are examined visibly for blood and volume but are discarded to eradicate gastric contents that might be affected by the stress of the intubation process. The patient is allowed no liquids during the test, and saliva must be ejected to avoid diluting the stomach contents.

The final four specimens collected during the test constitute the basal acid output. Each sample is titrated to pH 3.5 using 0.1 N sodium hydroxide. The millimoles of hydrogen ion in each sample are calculated from the amount of base used to neutralize the stomach acid of each. The results of the closest three samples are averaged and multiplied by four to give the millimoles of free hydrogen ions per hour. If analysis suggests abnormally low gastric secretion, the maximum acid output test is performed immediately afterward.

Gastric Acid Stimulation Test

After the basal samples have been collected, the tube remains in place for the gastric acid stimulation test. Pentagastrin, or a similar drug that stimulates gastric acid output, is injected subcutaneously. After 15 minutes, a specimen is collected every 15 minutes for one hour. These specimens are called the post-stimulation specimens. As is the case with the basal gastric secretion test, the patient can have no liquids during this test, and their saliva must be ejected to avoid diluting the stomach contents. The maximal acid output (MAO) is determined by titrating each of the four specimens and averaging the results. The average is used to determine the millimoles of hydrogen ion produced per hour. Alternatively, the peak acid output (PAO) is determined by titrating each specimen and using the average hydrogen ion concentration of the highest two to calculate the acid produced in millimoles per hour.

Analyses and Calculations

The appearance, blood, bile, pH, volume, millimoles of H+ per liter, millimoles of H+ per volume, and millimoles of free H+ per hour of each specimen are then evaluated. In addition, the basal acid output (BAO) is computed, as is the maximal acid output (MOA) or peak acid output (PAO). BAO is calculated by averaging the output of the three closest samples. MAO is calculated as the average of the four specimens. PAO is calculated by taking the mean of the two highest post-stimulation values.

There is a slight risk that the gastric tube may be inserted improperly, entering the trachea instead of the esophagus. If this happens, the patient may experience difficulty breathing or a coughing spell until the tube is correctly inserted. Also, because the tube can be difficult to swallow, if a patient has an overactive gag reflex, there may be a transient rise in blood pressure due to anxiety. Other complications may include bleeding, dysrhythmias, esophageal perforation, layrngospasm and decreased mean pO_2 (a measure of blood oxygen levels).

REFERENCES

Bandura, A. (1977). A social learning theory. Englewood Cliffs, NJ: Prentice Hall.

Bandura, A. (1986). Social foundation of thought and action: A social, cognitive theory. Englewood Cliffs, NJ: Prentice Hall.

Bartlik, B., Kocsis, J. H., & Legee, R. (1999). Sexual dysfunction secondary to depressive disorders. Journal of Sexual & Marital Therapy, 2(2), 52–60.

Burkhardt, M. A. (1993). Characteristics of spirituality in the lives of women in a rural Appalachian community. Journal of Transcultural Nursing, 4(2), 12–18.

Chapin, K. (1999). Probing the STDs. American Journal of Nursing, 99(7), 24AAA–24DDD).

Dossey, B., & Dossey, L. (1998). Attending to holistic care. American Journal of Nursing, 98(8), 35–38.

Dunn, H. (1961). High-level wellness. Arlington, VA: R. W. Beatty.

Edelman, C. & Mandle, C. L. (1997). Health promotion throughout the life span (4th ed.). St. Louis, Mosby-Yearbook.

Estes, M. E. (2001). Health assessment & physical examination (2nd ed.). Albany, NY: Delmar Publishers.

Giger, J. N. & Davidhizar, R. E. (1999). Transcultural nursing: Assessment and intervention (3rd ed.). St. Louis: Mosby–Yearbook.

Johnson, B. S. (1996). Psychiatric-mental health nursing: Adaptation and growth (4th ed.). Philadelphia: Lippincott.

14

Terminally Ill Patient

The rapid rise in the number of people suffering from terminally ill diseases pose particular problems for nurses, who are the group of healthcare workers most closely involved in their care. In contemporary society, individuals constantly experience loss. Frequent episodes of terrorism, natural disaster, and personal crises result in the universal experience of loss.

Throughout the life cycle, people are faced with loss, without which growth would not continue. Many people consider loss only in terms of death and dying; however, loss of every type occurs daily. Nurses must be aware of the potential for loss in today's world, as well as the processes by which individuals adapt. Every day nurses encounter clients who are responding to grief associated with losses. Thus, nurses must have an understanding of the major concepts related to loss and grieving. Grief is a response to losses of all types. Nurses also care for dying clients.

CONCEPTS OF LOSS, GRIEF, GRIEVING PROCESS

In contemporary society, persons constantly experience loss. Frequent episodes of terrorism, natural disaster, and personal crises result in the universal experience of loss. Throughout the life cycle, people are faced with loss, without which growth would not continue. Many people consider loss only in terms of death and dying; nevertheless, loss of every type occurs daily.

Nurses must be aware of the potential for loss in today's world, as well as the processes by which persons adapt. Every day nurses encounter clients who are responding to grief associated with losses. Thus, nurses must have an understanding of the major notions related to loss and grieving. Grief is a response to losses of all types.

LOSS

Loss is any situation (either actual, potential, or perceived) in which a valued object is changed or is no longer accessible to the individual. Because change is a major constant in life, everyone experiences losses. Loss can be actual (e.g., a spouse is lost through divorce) or anticipated (an individual is diagnosed with a terminal illness and has only a short time to live). A loss can be tangible or intangible. For instance, when an individual is fired from a job, the tangible loss is income, whereas the loss of self-esteem is intangible.

Loss precipitates anxiety and a feeling of vulnerability- which may lead to crisis. When a significant other dies, one's sense of safety and security is disrupted. Grieving is a mechanism for crisis resolution. When an individual feels overwhelmed by stress and the usual coping mechanisms are no longer effective, crisis occurs. Crisis intervention may be necessary to help the person grieve successfully. Loss occurs when a valued object is changed or is no longer available. Not everyone responds to loss in the same way because the significance of the lost object or person is determined by individual perceptions. There are many types of loss, including:

- Actual loss: Death of a loved one, theft of one's property
- Perceived loss: Occurs when a sense of loss is felt by an individual but is not tangible to others
- Physical loss: Loss of an extremity in an accident, scarring from burns, permanent injury
- Psychological loss: Such as a woman feeling inadequate after menopause and resultant infertility

Types of Loss

Loss of an Object: When an object that a person highly values is damaged, changed, or disappears, loss occurs. The significance of the lost object to the individual determines the type and amount of grieving that occurs. The valued object may be a person, pet, prized possession, or one's home. The loss of a pet, especially for those who live alone, can be a devastating loss.

Loss of Familiar Environment: The loss of a familiar environment occurs when a person moves to another home or a different community, changes schools, or starts a new job. Also, a client who is hospitalized or institutionalized experiences loss when faced with new surroundings. This type of loss evokes anxiety caused by fear of the unknown.

Loss of Self Aspect: Loss of an aspect of self can be physiological or psychological. A psychological aspect of self that may be lost is ambition, a sense of humour, or enjoyment of life. An example of physiological loss includes loss of physical function as a result of illness or injury. Loss also occurs when there is disfigurement or disappearance of a body part, such as having an amputation or mastectomy. Loss of an aspect of self can result from illness, trauma, or treatment methodologies.

Loss of loved one: The loss of a loved one is a significant loss. Such a loss can be the result of separation, divorce, running away, moving to a different area, or death. Responses to loss are highly individualized as each person perceives the meaning of loss differently. For example, the death of a spouse is different for men and women.

GRIEF

Grief is a series of intense physical and psychological responses that occur following a loss. It is a normal, natural, necessary, and adaptive response to a loss. Grieving is a walk through unknown territory. Familiar internal and external stabilities disappear in a whirlwind of changing thoughts, feelings, and emotional flux. Loss leads to the adaptive process of mourning, the period of time during which the grief is expressed and resolution and integration of the loss occur. Bereavement is the period of grief following the death of a loved one.

Resolution of a loss is a painful process and must be done by clients in their own way. Nurses can assist by providing support as the client moves through the process of mourning. Grief changes people by affecting self-esteem, triggering the development of new ways of coping, and precipitating a change in lifestyle without the deceased.

Types of Grief

Grief is a universal, normal response to loss. Grief drains people, both emotionally and physically. Because grief consumes so much emotional energy, relationships may be impaired and health status may become altered. There are different types of grief including uncomplicated ("normal"), dysfunctional, and anticipatory.

Uncomplicated Grief: Many individuals use the term normal grief. Engle proposed use of the term uncomplicated grief to describe a grief reaction that normally follows a significant loss. Uncomplicated grief runs a fairly predictable course that ends with the relinquishing of the lost object and resumption of the previous life. Of course, the bereaved person's life is changed forever, but the person is able to regain the ability to function. Not every mourner will experience all the reactions, but the reactions most often experienced in response to a recent loss are listed. Many grieving people experience feelings of anger or blame; these feelings may be directed toward those perceived to have caused or contributed to the death.

Often the anger associated with grief is directed at one's self, that is, expressed as guilt or depression. Some survivors have a strong need to assign blame. If someone else can be blamed, then the survivors can rid themselves of any responsibility. Those who are experiencing grief must be provided an opportunity to express feelings-both positive and negative-in order to alleviate guilt. Nurses play an important role in assisting mourners to develop and understand the normal grieving process and the complex feelings exhibited when grief becomes more complicated. Nurses with a sound knowledge base of both normal grief and dysfunctional grief will be better prepared to assist the survivors than nurses who believe that all grief is the same.

Dysfunctional Grief: Persons experiencing dysfunctional grief do not progress through the stages of overwhelming emotions associated with grief, or they may fail to demonstrate any behaviours commonly associated with grief. The person experiencing pathologic grief continues to have strong emotional reactions, does not return to a normal sleep pattern or work routine, usually remains isolated, and has altered eating habits. The bereaved may have the need to endlessly tell and retell the story of loss but without subsequent healing. The pathologically grieving person is unable to reestablish a routine. Dysfunctional grief is a demonstration of a persistent pattern of intense grief that does not result in reconciliation of feelings. A person experiencing chronic grief continues to focus on the deceased, may overvalue objects that belonged to the deceased, and may engage in depressive brooding.

DEATH

In today's social climate, death is viewed as something to be avoided at all costs; medicine, with its technological advances, pursues immortality. These scientific advances do not change the fact that death is a part of every human existence. No one expects to die. It is something that happens to someone else and to someone else's loved ones. Yet it is one of two life events that all humans share, the other being birth. Dying was once considered to be a normal part of the life cycle. Today it is often considered to be a medical problem that should be handled by health care providers. Technologic advances in medicine have caused care of those who are dying to become depersonalized and mechanical.

In an attempt to humanize care of the dying, proponents of improved EOL care are looking to nurses. Nurses spend more time with patients who are facing the end of life (EOL) than any other member of the health care team. This highly technologic world calls for application of high-touch intervention with the dying. In other words, appropriate care of the dying is administered by compassionate nurses who are both technically competent and able to demonstrate caring.

End-Of-Life (EOL) Care

No one expects to die. It is something that happens to someone else and to someone else's loved ones. Yet it is one of two life events that all humans share, the other being birth. Dying was once considered to be a normal part of the life cycle. Today it is often considered to be a medical problem that should be handled by health care providers. Technologic advances in medicine have caused care of those who are dying to become depersonalized and mechanical. In an attempt to humanize care of the dying, proponents of improved EOL care are looking to nurses. Nurses spend more time with patients who are facing the end of life (EOL) than any other member of the health care team. This highly technologic world calls for application of high-touch intervention with the dying. In other words, appropriate care of the dying is administered by compassionate nurses who are both technically competent and able to demonstrate caring.

A patient needs intensive physical and emotional support as he approaches death. Signs of impending death include reduced respiratory rate and depth, decreased or absent blood pressure, weak or erratic pulse rate, lowered skin temperature, decreased level of consciousness, diminished sensorium and neuromuscular control, diaphoresis, pallor, cyanosis, and mottling. Emotional support for the dying patient and his family most usually means reassurance and the nurse's physical presence to help ease fear and loneliness. More intense emotional support is significant at much earlier stages, especially for patients with long-term progressive illness who can work through the stages of dying. Respect the patient's wishes about extraordinary means of supporting life.

Stages of Dying

In her classic works, Elizabeth Kübler-Ross (1969, 1974) identified five possible stages of dying experienced by clients and their families. Every person does not move sequentially through each stage. These stages are experienced in varying degrees and for varying lengths of time. The client may express anger and, a few minutes later, express acceptance of the inevitable, then express anger again. The value in Kübler-Ross's work is that it helps increase sensitivity to the needs of the dying client.

Denial: In the first stage of dying, the initial shock can be overwhelming. Denial, which is an immediate response to loss experienced by most people, is a useful tool for coping. It is an essential and protective mechanism that may last for only a few minutes or may manifest itself for months.

Anger: The initial stage of denial is followed by anger. The client's security is being threatened by the unknown. All the normal daily routines have become disrupted. The client has no control over the situation and thus becomes angry in response to this powerlessness. The anger may be directed at self, God, and others. Often the nurse is the recipient of the anger when the client lashes out.

Bargaining: The anticipation of the loss through death brings about bargaining through which the client attempts to postpone or reverse the inevitable. The client promises to do something (such as be a better person, change lifestyle) in exchange for a longer life.

Depression: When the realization comes that the loss can no longer be delayed, the client moves to the stage of depression. This depression is different from dysfunctional depression in that it helps the client detach from life to be able to accept death.

Acceptance: The final stage of acceptance may not be reached by every dying client. However, "most dying persons eventually accept the inevitability of death. Many want to talk about their feelings with family members. Verbalization of emotions facilitates acceptance. With acceptance comes growing awareness of peace and contentment. The feeling that all that could be done has been done is often expressed during this stage. Reinforcement of the client's feelings and sense of personal worth are important during this stage.

CARE OF DEAD BODY

Caring for the deceased body and meeting the needs of the grieving family are nursing duties. The body of the deceased needs to be treated in a way that respects the sanctity of the human body. Nursing care includes maintaining privacy and preventing damage to the body.

Physiological Changes

Several physiological changes occur after death. The body temperature decreases with a resultant lack of skin elasticity (algor mortis). Therefore, the nurse must use caution when removing tape from the body to avoid skin breakdown. Another physiological change, liver mortis, is the bluish purple discolouration that is a byproduct of red blood cell destruction. This discolouration occurs in dependent areas of the body; hence, the nurse should elevate the head to prevent discolouration from the pooling of blood. Approximately 2 to 4 hours after death, rigor mortis occurs; this is stiffening of the body caused by contraction of skeletal and smooth muscles. To prevent disfiguring effects of rigor mortis, as soon as possible after death the nurse should close the eyelids, insert dentures (if applicable), close the mouth, and position the body in a natural position.

In preparing the body for family viewing, the nurse seeks to make the body look comfortable and natural.

This means removing all tubes and positioning the body as described. After the family has viewed the body, the nurse places identification tags on the body's toe and wrist. The body is then placed in a plastic or fabric shroud and the shroud is tagged. Then the body is transported to the morgue according to the agency's policy. The nurse is also accountable for returning the deceased's possessions to the family. Jewellery, eyeglasses, clothing, and all other personal items are returned to the family.

MEDICO-LEGAL ASPECTS

In most states, the physician is legally accountable for determining the cause of death and signing the death certificate. The nurse may, in certain situations, be the individual accountable for certifying the death. It is significant for nurses to know their legal duties, which are defined by their state or provincial board of nursing.

Organ Donation

The donation of organs for transplantation is a matter that requires compassion and sensitivity from the caregivers. Health care institutions are needed to have policies related to the referral of potential donors to organ procurement agencies. It is significant that families of the deceased know the significance of and process for organ donation. There is an inadequate supply of organs and tissues to meet the demand for transplants. The following organs and tissues are used for transplantation:

- Kidneys
- Heart
- Lungs
- Liver
- Pancreas
- Skin

- Corneas
- Bones (long bones and middle ear bones)

At the time the family gives consent for donation, the nurse notifies the donor team that an organ is available for transplant. Time is of the essence because the organ or tissue must be harvested and transplanted quickly to maintain viability.

AUTOPSY

An autopsy, also known as a post-mortem examination, necropsy (particularly as to animals), or obduction, is a medical procedure that comprises of a thorough examination of a corpse to determine the cause and manner of death and to evaluate any disease or injury that may be present. It is commonly performed by a specialized medical doctor called a pathologist.

Autopsies are either performed for legal or medical intentions. A forensic autopsy is carried out when the cause of death may be a criminal matter, while a clinical or academic autopsy is performed to find the medical cause of death and is used in cases of unknown or uncertain death, or for research intentions. Autopsies can be further classified into cases where external examination suffices, and those where the body is dissected and an internal examination is conducted. Permission from next of kin may be needed for internal autopsy in some cases. Once an internal autopsy is complete the body is reconstituted by sewing it back together.

EMBALMING

Embalming, in most modern cultures, is the art and science of temporarily preserving human remains to forestall decomposition and to make them suitable for display at a funeral. The three goals of embalming are thus preservation, sanitization and presentation (or restoration) of a dead body to achieve this effect. Embalming has a very long and cross-cultural history, with many cultures giving the embalming processes a greater religious meaning.

The first step in embalming is to check that the individual is in fact deceased, and then verify the identity of the body (typically via wrist or leg tags). At this point embalmers usually perform fundamental tests for signs of death, noting things such as clouded-over corneas, lividity, and rigor mortis or by simply attempting to palpate a pulse in the carotid or radial artery. In modern times people awakening on the preparation table is largely the province of horror fiction and urban myth. Any clothing on the corpse is removed and set aside and any personal effect such as jewellery is inventoried. A modesty cloth is sometimes placed over the genitalia. The corpse is washed in disinfectant and germicidal solutions. During this process the embalmer bends, flexes and massages the arms and legs to relieve rigor mortis.

The eyes are posed using an eye cap that keeps them shut and in the proper expression. The mouth may be closed via suturing with a needle and ligature, using an adhesive, or by setting a wire into the maxilla and mandible with a needle injector, a specialized device most usually utilized and unique to mortuary practice.

Care is taken to make the expression look as relaxed and natural as possible and ideally a recent photograph of the deceased while still living is used as a template. The process of closing the mouth, eyes, shaving, etc is collectively known as setting the features.

The actual embalming process commonly involves four parts:

1. Arterial embalming, which involves the injection of embalming chemicals into the blood vessels, commonly via the right common carotid artery. Blood is displaced from the right jugular vein. The embalming solution is injected with a centrifugal pump and the embalmer massages the corpse to break up circulatory clots as to ensure the proper distribution of the embalming fluid. In case of poor circulation, other injection points are used.
2. Cavity embalming, the suction of the internal fluids of the corpse and the injection of embalming chemicals into body cavities, using an aspirator and trocar. The embalmer makes a small incision just above the navel and pushes the trocar in the chest and stomach cavities to puncture the hollow organs and aspirate their contents. He then fills the cavities with concentrated chemicals that contain formaldehyde. The incision is either sutured closed or a "trocar button" is screwed into place.
3. Hypodermic embalming, the injection of embalming chemicals under the skin as required.
4. Surface embalming, which supplements the other methods, especially for visible, injured body parts.

A typical embalming takes one to two hours. An embalming case that requires more attention could take longer. The repair of an autopsy case or the restoration of a long-bone donor are two such examples.

REFERENCES

Aviramim, M., Ophir, R., Raviv, D., & Shiloah, M. (1999). Experiential learning of clinical skills by beginning nursing students. Journal of Nursing Education, 37(5), 228–231.

Bartling, A. C. (1995). Trends in managed care. Health Executive, 10(2), 6–11.

Bednash, G. (2000). The decreasing supply of registered nurses. Journal of the American Medical Association, 283(22), 2985–2989.

Braunstein, M. S. (1998). Evaluation of nursing practice: Process and critique. Nursing Science Quarterly, 11(2) 64–68.

Grady, P. A. (2000). News from NINR. Nursing Outlook, 48(1) 33.

Heggie, M., Melcher, P., & Williams, S. (1999). Hardiness, help-seeking, and social support of baccalaureate nursing students. Journal of Nursing Education, 38(4), 179–82.

Holm, K., & Llewellyn, J. G. (1986). Nursing research for nursing practice. Philadelphia: Saunders.

Hynes, D. M. (2000). Research as a key to promoting and sustaining innovate practice. Nursing Clinics of North America, 35(2), 453–459.

Lenz, E. R. (1994). Paradigm shifts, changing contexts, and graduate nursing education. In A changing health care system. Atlanta, GA: Southern Council on Collegiate Education for Nursing.

Hewlett, P., & Eichelberger, L. (1996). The case against mandatory continuing education. Journal of Continuing Education in Nursing, 27(4), 176–181.

15

Nursing Concepts & Theories

Nursing theory is the term given to the body of knowledge that is used to support nursing practice. In their professional education nurses will study a range of interconnected subjects which can be applied to the practice setting. This knowledge may be derived from experiential learning, from formal sources such as nursing research or from non-nursing sources. To speak of nursing theory is often difficult. Nursing is many things to many people. Most universally agreed upon is that Nursing is a science involving people, environment and process fuelled by a vision of transcendence in the context of healthcare. It is interesting to note that 90% of all Nursing theories have been generated in the last 20 years. Many schools encourage students to formulate personal philosophies or mid-range theories of Nursing as part of their curriculum. Some might argue that this multiplicity of theory is detrimental to the practice and undermines common vision. Others would say that the nature of the young science is sufficiently far reaching to require such tactics in order to elicit true consensus.

Nursing models are conceptual models, constructed of theories and concepts. They are used to help nurses assess, plan, and implement patient care by providing a framework within which to work. They also help nurses achieve uniformity and seamless care.

UNIVERSAL FEATURES OF NURSING MODELS

Unlike most sciences, Nursing theories seem primarily concerned with what "Nursing" is or should do, rather than a phenomenon of Nursing". All nursing models involve some method of evaluating a patient's individual needs and implementing appropriate patient care. An essential portion of each nursing model is measurable goals in order that the process can be evaluated in order to provide better, is used to determine a patient's treatment by nurses, doctors and other healthcare professionals and auxiliary workers. These documents are considered to be living documents - they are changed and evaluated on a daily basis as the patients condition an abilities change.

NURSING MODELS

The original role of the nurse was primarily to care for the patient as prescribed by a physician. This evolved into the biomedical model of nursing care which still strongly influences nursing practice today. The biomedical model focuses heavily upon pathophysiology and altered homeostasis but fails to identify individual differences and whilst it works well for traditional medical and physical care, it focuses solely on the treatment of disease, making little account of psychological, social, cultural, and economic differences between persons. The Biomedical Model essentially views all patients with the same disease as the same problem regardless of their religion, culture, or ethnicity. This is in contrast to the social model of healthcare that places emphasis on changes that can be made in society and in people's own lifestyles to make the population healthier.

The first theorist to clearly articulate a role of nurses distinct from the medical profession was Florence Nightingale. Her theories were developed during the Crimean War and published in Notes on Nursing: What It Is, and What It Is Not in 1859. Nightingale's model is based on the idea that the nurse manipulates the environment to promote the patient's well-being. Nurses quickly realised that treating patients based upon their disease rather than making a holistic evaluation was not a satisfactory way of attending patient care.

THEORIES IN NURSING

Nursing has made phenomenal achievement in the last century that has lead to the recognition of nursing as an academic discipline and a profession. A move towards theory-based practice has made contemporary nursing more meaningful and significant by shifting nursing's focus from vocation to an organised profession. The need for knowledge-base to guide professional nursing practice had been realised in the first half of the twentieth century and many theoretical works have been contributed by nurses ever since, first with the goal of making nursing a recognised profession and later with the goal of delivering care to patients as professionals.

A theory is a group of related notions that propose action that guide practice. A nursing theory is a set of notions, definitions, relationships, and assumptions or propositions derived from nursing models or from other disciplines and project a purposive, systematic view of phenomena by designing specific inter-relationships among notions for the intentions of describing, explaining, predicting, and /or prescribing..

Based on the knowledge structure levels the theoretical works in nursing can be studied under the following headings:

- Metaparadigm (Person, Environment, Health & Nursing) - (Most abstract)
- Nursing philosophies.
- Conceptual models and Grand theories.
- Nursing theories and Middle range theories (Least abstract)

The conceptual and theoretical nursing models help to provide knowledge to improve practice, guide research and curriculum and identify the goals of nursing practice. The state of art and science of nursing theory is one of continuing growth. Using the internet the nurses of the world can share ideas and knowledge, carrying on the work begun by nursing theorists and continue the growth and development of new nursing knowledge. It is significant the nursing knowledge is learnt, used, and applied in the theory based practice for the profession and the continued development of nursing and academic discipline

PEPLAU'S THEORY

Peplau (1952) described nursing as "a significant, therapeutic, interpersonal process. It functions co-operatively with other human processes that make health possible for persons in communities. Nursing is an educative instrument, a maturing force, that aims to promote forward movement of personality in the direction of creative, constructive, productive, personal and community living". Lack of growth, for whatever reason, implies impaired health in the individual and fundamental human needs must be met if a fit state is to be achieved and maintained.

A number of assumptions are implicit in Peplau's original and latter writings. For instance, the relationship of nurse and patient is influential in the outcome for the patient; People may assume a number of roles and have the capacity for empathy in relationships; People tend to behave in ways which have worked in the past when faced with a crisis; Anxiety and tension arise from unmet or conflicting needs, and the energy which arises may be harnessed into positive means for defining, understanding and meeting the problem at hand.

The nurse patient relationship is characterised by a number of overlapping phases with a number of therapeutic tasks or goals to be accomplished. During each phase the patient expresses needs which find expression and require intervention in unique ways.

Orientation Phase: The phase of the relationship, when the nurse and patient first meet is known as the orientation phase. This is a time when the patient and nurse come to know each other as people and each other's expectations and roles are understood. The patient at this time needs to recognise and understand their difficulty and the need for help, be assisted to plan to use the professional services offered, and harness the energy derived from felt needs. It may be expected that the patient will test limits in order to establish the integrity of the nurse. The tasks of this phase are to build trust, rapport, establish a therapeutic environment, evaluate the patients strengths and weakness and establish a mode of communication acceptable to both patient and nurse. When the patient can begin to identify problems the relationship progresses to the working phase.

Working Phase: The working phase incorporates the identification and exploitation sub-phases and the relationship may fluctuate back and forth as new problems are identified. During the identification phase trust begins to develop and the patient begins to respond selectively to persons who seem to offer help. The patient begins to identify with the nurse and identify problems, which can be worked on. The meaning behind feelings and behaviour of the nurse and patient are explored. Peplau states that when a nurse permits patients to express what they feel, and still get all of the nursing that is required, then patients can undergo illness as an experience that reorients feelings and strengthens positive forces in the personality. The tasks of this phase are to develop clarity about the patient's preconceptions and expectations of nurses and nursing, develop acceptance of each other, explore feelings, identify problems and respond to people who can offer help. In particular the nurse assists in the expression of needs and feelings, assists during stress, shows acceptance and provides information. The nurse and patient may make plans for the future but the implementation of the plan signifies the beginning of the exploitation phase of the working relationship.

During the exploitation phase the patient realistically exploits all of the services available to them on the basis of self interest and need. The nurse assists the patient in their efforts to strike a balance between the needs for dependence and independence. The plan of action is implemented and evaluated. The patient may display a change in manner of communicating, as new skills in interpersonal relationships and problem solving are developed. The nurse continues to evaluate and assists in meeting new needs as they emerge.

Resolution Phase: The resolution phase involves the gradual freeing from identification with helping persons, and the generation and strengthening of ability to stand alone, eventually leading to the mutual termination of the relationship. The patient abandons old needs and aspires to new goals. She or he continues to apply new problem solving skills and maintains changes in style of communication and interaction. Resolution includes planning for alternative sources of support, problem prevention, and the patient's integration of the illness experience.

HENDERSON'S THEORY

The Henderson theory of nursing covers a definition of nursing, a description of the function of a nurse, and the enumeration of the 14 components that make up fundamental nursing care.

The Henderson theory of nursing was developed by Virginia Henderson. She didn't believe that she was setting out a theory, and preferred it to be thought of as a definition. Whether it is considered a definition or a theory, it has had a wide influence on concept and practice of nursing.

The definition of nursing is the fundamental part of Henderson's theory of nursing. Henderson defined nursing as doing things for patients that they would do for themselves if they could, that is if they were physically able or had the needed knowledge. Nursing helps the patient become fit or die peacefully, and also helps people work toward independence, so that they can begin to perform the relevant activities for themselves as quickly as possible. Rather than focus on a particular task, Henderson focused on the patient. She saw how nursing could focus on the patient, and how it was possible to focus on developing a good nurse-patient relationship. This deeply affected her and she believed strongly that patient-focused nursing was the most beneficial kind of nursing for the patient.

Henderson also enumerated the 14 functions she believed to be part of fundamental nursing care. The nurse should help the patient to perform the following functions:

- Eat and drink
- Breathe
- Move
- Sleep
- Dress
- Work to gain a sense of accomplishment
- Maintain normal body temperature
- Eliminate wastes
- Keep clean
- Communicate
- Participate in recreation
- Worship
- Avoid dangers or hurting others
- Learn and discover

When the patient was able to perform all the functions by him or herself then the patient could be considered independent and no longer needed the aid of a nurse.

Virginia Henderson also believed that it was significant that nursing be based on evidence, and that research was a critical component of improving nursing practice. She believed all nurses should have access to literature on nursing and current nursing research to help better their practices, and to this end, she worked to develop an index of nursing. Virginia Henderson played a very significant role in the development of modern nursing. Her contributions, especially to evidence based nursing practice, are considered so significant that Sigma Theta Tau's International Nursing Library has been named in her honour.

OREM'S THEORY

The Orem model of nursing was developed between 1959 and 2001 by Dorothea Orem and is also known as the 'Self Care' Model of Nursing. It is particularly used in rehabilitation and primary care settings where the patient is encouraged to be as independent as possible. The Orem model is based upon the philosophy that all "patients wish to care for themselves".

Self care Requisites: Self care requisites are groups of needs or requirements that Orem identified. They are classified as either:

- Universal self care requisites - those needs that all people have
- Developmental self care requisites - those needs that relate to development of the individual
- Health deviation requisites - those needs that arise as a result of a patient's condition

Self care deficits: When an individual is very unable to meet their own Self care requisites, a Self Care Deficit occurs. It is the job of the Registered Nurse to determine these deficits, and define a support modality.

Support modalities: Nurses are encouraged to rate their patient's dependencies or each of the self care deficits on the following scale:

- Total Compensation
- Partial Compensation
- Educative/Supportive

Universal Self Care Requisites (SCRs): The Universal self care requisites that all or health are:

- Air
- Water
- Food
- Elimination
- Activity and Rest
- Solitude and Social Interaction
- Hazard Prevention
- Promotion of Normality

The nurse is encouraged to assign a support modality to each of the self care requisites.

NEUMAN'S THEORY OF NURSING

The Neuman Systems Model provides a comprehensive, system based conceptual framework. Originally designed to be used in nursing it can be used by other health professions. The intention of the model is to provide a unifying focus for approaching a wide range of nursing concerns and for understanding fundamental nursing phenomena: the client, the environment, health and nursing.

The model represents the client within the system perspective, wholistically and multi-dimensionally. It shows the components of five interacting client variables; physiological, psychological, developmental, sociocultural and spiritual in relation to environmental influences upon the client as a system consisting of fundamental structure, lines of resistance and lines of defence.

The environment is broadly defines all internal and external factors or influences surrounding the identified client or client system. Environment comprises of three dimensions: internal environment, external environment and created environment.

The health of the client is envisioned as being at various levels within a normal range, rising or falling throughout the life span related to adjustment by the client system to environmental stressors.

The major concern of nursing is keeping the client system stable throughout constant life changes with accuracy both in evaluating the effects of environmental stressors and in assisting client adjustments needed for optimal level wellness through primary, secondary and tertiary prevention strategies as intervention.

ROYS' THEORY

Assumptions

Scientific

- Systems of matter and energy progress to higher levels of complex self-organization
- Consciousness and meaning are constitutive of individual and environment integration
- Awareness of self and environment is rooted in thinking and feeling
- Humans by their decisions are responsible for the integration of creative processes
- Thinking and feeling mediate human action
- System relationships include acceptance, protection, and fostering of interdependence
- Persons and the earth have common patterns and integral relationships
- Persons and environment transformations are created in human consciousness
- Integration of human and environment meanings results in adaptation

Philosophical

- Persons have mutual relationships with the world and God
- Human meaning is rooted in an omega point convergence of the universe
- God is intimately revealed in the diversity of creation and is the common destiny of creation
- Persons use human creative abilities of awareness, enlightenment, and faith
- Persons are responsible for the processes of deriving, sustaining, and transforming the universe

Environment

- All conditions, circumstances, and influences surrounding and affecting the development and behaviour of persons and groups with particular consideration of mutuality of individual and earth resources
- Three kinds of stimuli: focal, contextual, and residual
- Significant stimuli in all human adaptation include stage of development, family, and culture

Health and Adaptation

- Health: a state and process of being and becoming integrated and whole that reflects individual and environmental mutuality
- Adaptation: the process and outcome whereby thinking and feeling persons, as persons and in groups, use conscious awareness and choice to create human and environmental integration
- Adaptive Responses: responses that promotes integrity in terms of the goals of the human system, that is, survival, growth, reproduction, mastery, and personal and environmental transformation
- Ineffective Responses: responses that do not contribute to integrity in terms of the goals of the human system
- Adaptation levels represent the condition of the life processes described on three different levels: integrated, compensatory, and compromised

Nursing

- Nursing is the science and practice that expands adaptive abilities and develops individual and environment transformation
- Nursing goals are to promote adaptation for persons and groups in the four adaptive modes, thus contributing to health, quality of life, and dying with dignity
- This is done by evaluating behaviour and factors that influence adaptive abilities and by intervening to expand those abilities and to develop environmental interactions

Nursing Process

- A problem solving approach for gathering data, identifying the capacities and needs of the human adaptive system, selecting and implementing approaches for nursing care and assessment.
- Assessment of Behaviour: the first step of the nursing process which involves gathering data about the behaviour of the individual as an adaptive system in each of the adaptive modes
- Assessment of Stimuli: the second step of the nursing process which involves the identification of internal and external stimuli that are influencing the person's adaptive behaviours. Stimuli are classified as: (1) Focal- those most immediately confronting the person; (2) Contextual-all other stimuli present that are affecting the situation and (3) Residual- those stimuli whose effect on the situation are unclear.
- Nursing Diagnosis: step three of the nursing process which involves the formulation of statements that interpret data about the adaptation status of the person, including the behaviour and most relevant stimuli
- Goal Setting: the forth step of the nursing process which involves the establishment of clear statements of the behavioural outcomes for nursing care.
- Intervention: the fifth step of the nursing process which involves the determination of how best to assist the individual in attaining the established goals
- Evaluation: the sixth and final step of the nursing process which involves judging the effectiveness of the nursing intervention in relation to the behaviour after the nursing intervention in comparison with the goal established.

PURPOSES OF NURSING THEORY IN NURSING EDUCATION, RESEARCH, AND CLINICAL PRACTICE

In the early part of nursing's history, knowledge was extremely limited and almost entirely task oriented. The knowledge explosion that occurred in health care in the 1950s produced the need to systematically organize the tremendous volume of new information being generated. From the very beginnings of nursing education, there was a need to categorize knowledge and to analyze client care situations in order to communicate in coherent and meaningful ways. The literature about the relationship between theory and nursing care yields many interpretations in terms of the role each component plays in the health care environment. According to Barnum, "a theory is a construct that accounts for or organizes some phenomenon."

In addition, nursing theories provide a structure for communicating with other nurses and with other members of the healthcare team. Nursing theories assist the discipline of nursing in clarifying beliefs, values, and goals, and they help to define the unique contribution of nursing in the care of clients. When the focus of nursing's contribution is clear, then greater professional autonomy and, ultimately, control of certain aspects of practice are achieved. In the broadest sense, nursing theory is necessary for the continued development and evolution of the discipline of nursing. Because the world of health care changes virtually on a daily basis, nursing needs to continue to expand its knowledge base to proactively respond to changes in societal needs. Knowledge for nursing practice is developed through nursing research that, in turn, is used to either test existing theories or generate new theories. Nursing research is the systematic application of formalized methods for generating valid and dependable information about the phenomena of concern to the discipline of nursing.

COMPONENTS OF THE METAPARADIGM FOR NURSING

The metaparadigm of a discipline identifies common areas of concern. A paradigm is a particular way of viewing the phenomena of concern that have been delineated by the metaparadigm of the discipline. The term paradigm stems from the work of Kuhn, who referred to a paradigm as "worldview" about the phenomena of concern in a discipline. Two individuals with different paradigmatic views can look at precisely the same phenomenon and each will "see" or view the phenomenon differently. For instance, consider the viewpoints of a mother and father who are watching their daughter at T-ball practice. The mother looks at her daughter and "sees" a graceful, yet somewhat shy child who has shown improvement in her ability to make new friends. On the other hand, the father" sees" a strong runner who needs help with batting drills. Each parent is looking at the same phenomenon (their daughter), but each is "seeing" the phenomenon from a completely different perspective.

Each parent is operating from a different paradigm. The prevailing paradigm in a discipline represents the dominant viewpoint of particular concepts. This viewpoint is supported by theories and research that for the time being adequately address the concerns of the discipline. By consensus, the community of scholars in discipline accepts and agrees on a particular viewpoint or worldview. When new theories and research surface that challenge the prevailing paradigm, a new paradigm emerges to compete with the prevailing worldview. The competition between the paradigms results in what Kuhn (1970) refers to as a paradigm revolution. A paradigm revolution is the turmoil and conflict that occur in a discipline when a competing paradigm gains acceptance over the dominant paradigm. If the competing paradigm answers more questions and solves more problems for the discipline than the prevailing paradigm, then a paradigm shift occurs. A paradigm shift refers to the acceptance of the competing paradigm over the prevailing paradigm or a shifting away from one worldview toward another worldview.

LINKING THEORIES WITH NURSING PROCESS

Strategies for combining theory and diagnoses include emphasizing the diagnostic terms as professional shorthand and permitting flexibility in modifying diagnoses as required; widely disseminating the concept that classification can be used effectively with newer iterations of the nursing process reflecting circular, simultaneous, and intuitive processes; developing classification language based on concepts of hypothesis and perception; and including diagnostic categories associated with theoretical perspectives. Theory provides nurses with a perspective with which to view client situations, a way to organize the hundreds of data bits encountered in the day-to-day care of clients, and a way to analyze and interpret the information.

There is no question that use of nursing diagnosis, classification systems, and theory has enhanced the degree to which nurses are able to identify nursing work as significant, visible, and separate from the work of others. Despite the cited benefits of use of both theory and diagnosis, nevertheless, theorists eschew the use of nursing diagnosis, claiming the superiority of theory-derived language and philosophic bases that are incompatible with nursing diagnostic categorization. The intentions of this article are to articulate the philosophic and paradigmatic underpinnings of currently used theories, and to pose strategies for developing and integrating the language of nursing classification and theory in a way that will accommodate the conceptual perspectives of the theories.

There are significant values and assumptions about nursing practice that inhibit the simultanéous use of theory and diagnosis. It is imperative that those interested in nursing classifications address these values and assumptions and work to understand the perspectives of those who use the classifications and those who do not.

Outcomes of nursing care must be shown to relate to specific aspects of care provided. This relating of outcome to care can be done and evaluated only in the presence of classification terms or labels. It is incumbent on classifiers to reach out to capture the richness that is nursing in all of its theoretical perspectives. It is time for adherents of theories to use tools needed for research, evidence-based practice, and documentation and reimbursement of care. The two groups must "co-create" a system of classification that will best meet the professional needs of nursing as a whole.

EFFECTS OF USING THEORY TO UNDERSTAND CLINICAL PRACTICE

Current theorists are continually expanding and refining the work of theorists before them, and they are developing new ways of looking at the metaparadigm concepts of person, environment, health, and nursing. Our understanding of the nature of nursing is, and always has been, in a state of change. Though change is healthy and leads to growth, it is not always easy. Knowledge is not static, and what one learns today maybe challenged by different thoughts tomorrow. The world of health care changes on a daily basis. Client needs and problems often change on a minute by-minute basis. Knowledge, information, and technology in both health care and nursing are growing at unprecedented rates. In the face of these advances, nursing strives to preserve the notion of caring in healthcare.

Theories are needed to organize knowledge and to guide nursing practice and nursing research. More nursing research is needed to confirm or refute theories. A strong theoretical foundation on which to base the practice of nursing is essential. Nurses encounter a variety of clinical situations in which application of nursing theory is needed. In these occurrences, nurses may discover that specific theories will be more appropriate for certain clinical situations than others. Knowledge of specific theories should expand as nurses gain experience in nursing practice. In all cases, theories that are selected for application in practice should be congruent with the nurse's own beliefs and values.

REFERENCES

Fawcett, J. (1989). Analysis and evaluation of conceptual models of nursing (2nd ed.). Philadelphia: F. A. Davis.

Fawcett, J., (1993). Analysis and evaluation of nursing theories. Philadelphia: F. A. Davis.

Fawcett, J., Tulman, J., & Spedden, J. P. (1994). Responses to vaginal birth after cesarean section. Journal of Obstetric, Gynecologic and Neonatal Nursing, 23(3), 253–259.

Fitzpatrick, J. J. (1989). A life perspective rhythm model. In J. J. Fitzpatrick & A. Whall (Eds.), Conceptual models of nursing (2nd ed.). East Norwalk, CT: Appleton & Lange.

Kuhn, T. (1970). The Structure of scientific revolutions (2nd ed.). Chicago: The University of Chicago Press.

Levine, M. (1989). The four conservation principles: 20 years later. In J. Riehl-Sisca (Ed.), Conceptual models for nursing practice (3rd ed.). Stamford, CT: Appleton & Lange.

Rogers, M. (1990). Nursing: Science of unitary, irreducible human beings: Update 1990. In E. Barrett (Ed.), Visions of Rogers' science based nursing. New York: National League for Nursing.

Watson, J. (1985). Nursing: Human science and human care. Norwalk, CT: Appleton-Century-Crofts.

Yamashita, M. (1999) Newman's theory of health applied in family caregiving in Canada. Nursing Science Quarterly, 12(1), 73–79.

16

Legal Aspects

The word law is derived from an Anglo-Saxon term meaning that which is laid down or fixed. The two types of law are: public law, which deals with an individual's relationship to the state, and civil law, which deals with relations between persons.

Medical malpractice is said to be taking place when a medical practitioner is acting in a negligent manner while undertaking treatment of some medical condition. The medical malpractice law is a branch of personal injury law. This deals with pain and suffering caused owing to some gross mistake(s), negligence or bad judgment on the part of a doctor or other medical practitioner.

Failure to diagnose or wrongly diagnose a disease or medical condition, failure to provide right treatment for the condition and unreasonable delay in treating a medical condition diagnosed are common examples of medical malpractice that are sought to be redressed by enforcement of medical malpractice law.

The roots of the medical malpractice law can be traced back to the nineteenth century English common law. The general law body dealing with injuries to people or property- the tort law included the laws that developed concerning medical malpractices.

PURPOSE AND ESSENTIAL ELEMENTS OF INFORMED CONSENT

Laws regarding informed consent protect the client's right to self-determination. A client is able to make an informed decision about consenting to or refusing a treatment regime only if adequate information has been presented. The law requires that clients or their representatives be given sufficient information regarding various treatment modalities so that the consent is an informed process. Consent is a voluntary act by which a person agrees to allow someone else to do something. Informed consent means that the client understands the reason for the proposed intervention, and its benefits and risks, and agrees to the treatment by signing a consent form.

Consent forms must be obtained for all invasive (accessing body tissues, organs, or cavities through some type of instrumentation) procedures. Legally the client must be mentally competent to give consent for medical procedures.

When the nurse discovers circumstances that render a signed consent form invalid (such as a change in the client's condition) the nurse should notify the physician. If the client will not be harmed by a delay, the nurse is justified in refusing to assist with a procedure until the requirements for the informed consent are satisfied. Though the law does not require staff nurses to obtain a formal informed consent for nursing procedures, the nurse has the duty of explaining to the client what to expect during the procedure.

NURSE'S LEGAL RESPONSIBILITIES WITH SELECTED ASPECTS OF NURSING PRACTICE

A significant principle to live by in avoiding malpractice lawsuits is sharing the legal duty whenever possible. Nursing decisions are made every day by nurses in regards to patient care. In most instances, these patient care decisions are based on each nurse's professional experience and judgment; for instance, when a blood pressure reading is beyond the normal range for a patient and the nurse, in most cases, decides how to respond and treat this phenomenon without consulting a colleague or physician.

However, in certain situations it is imperative to share the legal duty. For instance, a patient takes a sudden and unexpected turn for the worse in a cardiac unit. It is necessary to immediately inform the physician of this change; nevertheless, the physician is unavailable or does not return a page or phone call. Does the nurse just wait until the physician responds? What if the patient continues to worsen despite attempts to stabilize. Here is an example of a situation in which sharing the legal duty will not only assist the nurse, but it will meet the standard of care for the patient.

Sharing the legal duty simply means discussing the situation with your immediate supervisor, who can assist in the decision-making process; in other words, "go up the chain of command." If the appropriate response is not forthcoming, continue to go up the chain of command. Remember, your duty is first and foremost to the patient

Other avenues of sharing the legal duty can be remembered on a vertical and/or horizontal plane. Going up the chain of command is to go up the vertical plane. Do not forget that assistance and consensus can be received from others who may have less duty than you. For instance, if you are a the supervising nurse of the unit, the primary care nurse reporting to you may be the appropriate individual to assist in making a decision or discussion a course of action. On a horizontal plane, any of your colleagues or allied healthcare professionals, such as physical therapists, could be the appropriate party to discuss a course of action. When the quality of patient care is compromised, it is best to discuss and share the duty with others. Making a decision entirely on your own is the quickest way to be named as a defendant in a malpractice lawsuit. Imagine having to testify that you knew the quality of patient of care had been compromised yet you discussed this with no one or asked for any assistance. The entire weight of the lawsuit could rest on your shoulders.

In addition to the professional staff, involving the patient and the patient's family is a significant part of the decision-making process. It is less likely that you will be found guilty of malpractice if the patient and his or her family were involved and had full disclosure of the situation.

All these discussions and courses should be fully documented. Do not rely on your memory to recall these significant conversations. As we have discussed earlier, documentation is the most significant tool in your arsenal to avoid malpractice lawsuits.

DIFFERENCE BETWEEN NEGLIGENCE AND MALPRACTICE

When the nurse fails to meet the legal expectations of care, the client can initiate action if harm or injury is incurred by the client. Liability is an obligation one has incurred or might incur through any act or failure to act. The term malpractice refers to the behaviour of a professional person's wrongful conduct, improper discharge of professional responsibilities, or failure to meet the standards of acceptable care, which result in harm to another individual. Negligence (breach of duty) is the failure of an individual to provide care that a reasonable individual would ordinarily use in a similar circumstance. In other words, action that is contrary to the conduct of a reasonable individual and results in harm is considered to be negligent behaviour. When a nurse commits a negligent act that results in injury, it is known as malpractice. Proof of liability depends on four elements:

1. Duty is an obligation created either by law or contractor by any voluntary action. It is the first element that must be proved for malpractice as it arises from the nurse-client relationship.
2. Breach of duty occurs when a nurse fails to act in accord with the standard of care. An act of commission or omission of the nurse may constitute a breach of the standard of care.
3. Injury (physical, financial, or emotional harm) must be demonstrated by the individual making the claim to prove negligence. Damages are the money or other compensation awarded by the court to the plaintiff (the party who initiates a lawsuit that seeks damages or other relief).
4. Causation is the breach of duty that must be proved to have legally caused the injury. A cause-and-effect relationship must be clearly established. To succeed in a malpractice suit, the plaintiff must first show that the defendant (the individual being sued) owed him a duty. The plaintiff must then show that the defendant didn't meet the duty and that this breach of duty caused harm, requiring compensation. Once the plaintiff files charges, the defendant must either refute the charges by demonstrating that, if a duty was owed, the duty was fulfilled or that, if a duty was breached, the breach was not the cause of the plaintiff's complaint of injury.

PROFESSIONAL LIABILITY INSURANCE

Professional liability insurance, also called Professional Indemnity Insurance, protects professional practitioners such as architects, lawyers, physicians, and accountants against potential negligence claims made by their patients/clients. Professional liability insurance may take on different names depending on the profession. For instance, professional liability insurance in reference to the medical profession may be called Medical Malpractice. Notaries public may take out errors and omissions insurance (E&O). Other potential E&O policyholders include, for instance, real estate brokers, home inspectors, appraisers, and website developers.

There are also specific E&O policies for technology companies, such as software developers, technology consultants and other creators of technology. This coverage focuses on the failure to perform, financial loss and error or omission of the products or services sold. Additional coverage for breach of warranty, intellectual property, personal injury, security and cost of contract can be added. The primary reason for professional liability coverage is that a typical general liability insurance policy will only respond to a bodily injury, property damage, personal injury or advertising injury claim. The above mentioned professional services and products can cause claims without causing a bodily injury, property damage, personal injury or advertising injury.

Common reasons alleged in making claims on these policies are negligence, misrepresentation, violation of good faith and fair dealing, and inaccurate advice. For instance, if a software product fails to perform correctly, it may not cause physical damages, personal or advertising injuries, hence the general liability policy would not be triggered. It may, nevertheless, directly cause financial losses which could potentially be attributed to the software developer's misrepresentation of the product capabilities. Professional liability insurance policies are generally set up based on a claims-made basis, meaning that the policy only covers incidents that occurred during the timeframe in which the coverage was active. It is significant to continue your coverage, because cancelling the policy, will in effect, make it as if you never had coverage.

DIFFERENT WAYS TO MINIMIZE CHANCES OF LIABILITY

There is a common set of actions a nurse can take to protect against litigation. Though each client encountered presents unique situations that can place the nurse at legal risk, certain general nursing care activities decrease this risk. Following the rules in the checklist should help protect nurses from lawsuits as well as provide defence in the event of a suit. All health care facilities have policies. Nursing students and registered nurses are obligated to know the policies and follow the procedures/protocols that flow from policy. Though policies are not laws, courts generally rule against nurses who violate policies.

Nurses should consider purchasing their own liability insurance for protection against malpractice lawsuits. Nurses may erroneously assume that they are protected by their employer's professional liability policies. When securing liability insurance, the nurse should validate the company's reputation. Most professional nursing organizations offer group liability insurance. Commonly when a nurse is sued, the employer is also sued for the nurse's actions or inaction. Although this is the norm, nurses are encouraged to have their own malpractice insurance. For instance, a suit may be filed for an incident that occurred in a facility where the nurse is no longer employed. Having one's own insurance also provides the nurse protection as an individual and allows the nurse to have an attorney who has only the nurse's interests in mind. Risk management is a method of identifying, assessing, and decreasing the agency's risk of financial loss.

Most health care facilities are needed to have formal risk management programs in place by agencies such as the Department of Health and Human Services, accrediting bodies, and liability insurance carriers. These programs are based on systematic reporting of incidents or unusual occurrences, for instance, client falls. In accord with the agency's policies, nurses are required to file incident reports when a situation arises that could or did cause client harm. When filing an incident report, the nurse should state only the facts surrounding the incident. The nurse's opinions or conclusions about the incident are not to be documented. Also, the client's medical record should not contain any reference to the filing of an incident report.

REFERENCES

Andrews, M. M., & Boyle, J. S. (1998). Transcultural concepts in nursing care (3rd ed.). Philadelphia: Lippincott.

Callister, L. C., Semenic, S., & Foster, J. C. (1999). Cultural and spiritual meanings of childbirth: Orthodox Jewish and Mormon women. Journal of Holistic Nursing, 17(3), 280–294.

Camphinha-Bacote, J. (1999). A model and instrument of addressing cultural competence in health care. Journal of Nursing Education, 38(5), 203–207. Centers for Disease Control and Prevention. (1998).

Edelman, C. L., & Mandle, C. L. (1997). Health promotion throughout the life span (4th ed.). St. Louis: Mosby- Yearbook.

Fralic, M. F. (1995). Leading a diverse healthcare workforce [Comment]. Capsules & Comments in Nursing Leadership & Management, 2(4), 31.

Geissler, E. M. (1998). Pocket guide to cultural assessment. New York: Times Mirror.

Giger, J. N. & Davidhizar, R. E. (1998). Canadian transcultural nursing: Assessment and intervention. St. Louis: Mosby.

Giger, J. N., & Davidhizar, R. E. (1999). Transcultural nursing: Assessment and intervention (3rd ed.). St. Louis: Mosby-Yearbook.

Bibliography

Ackley, B. J., & Ladwig, G. B. (1997). Nursing diagnostic handbook (3rd ed.). St. Louis: Mosby Year-Book.

Adams, E. (1983). Frontiers of nursing in the 21st century: Development of models and theories on the concept of nursing. Journal of Advanced Nursing, 8, 41-45.

Aiken, L. H. (1995). Transformation of the nursing workforce. Nursing Outlook, 43(5), 201-209.

Andrews, M. M., & Boyle, J. S. (1998). Transcultural concepts in nursing care (3rd ed.). Philadelphia: Lippincott.

Bartling, A. C. (1995). Trends in managed care. Health Executive, 10(2), 6-11.

Benner, P., & Wrubel, J. (1988). Caring comes first. American Journal of Nursing, 8(4), 1072-1075.

Bevis, E. O. (1989). Curriculum building in nursing: A process (3rd ed., Publication No. 15-2277). New York: National League for Nursing.

Carpenito, L. J. (1999). Nursing diagnosis: Application to clinical practice (7th ed.). Philadelphia: Lippincott.

Carper, B. A. (1978). Fundamental patterns of knowing in nursing. Advances in Nursing Science, 1, 13-23.

Collins, A. M., & Diego, L. (2000). Mental health promotion and protection. Journal of Psychosocial Nursing, 38(1), 27-32.

Crellin, K. (1998). 11 easy ways to build rapport. Nursing98, November 28(11): 48-49.

Doenges, M. E., & Moorhouse, M. F. (1995). Application of nursing process and nursing diagnosis (2nd ed.). Philadelphia: F. A. Davis.

Economic Policy Institute. (1999). Sharing care: The changing nature of nursing. Washington, DC: Author.

Fawcett, J., (1993). Analysis and evaluation of nursing theories. Philadelphia: F. A. Davis.

Feldstein, P. J. (1993). Health care economics (4th ed.). Albany, NY: Delmar Publishers.

Gordan, R. C. (1999). Linda Richards at the Kalamazoo State Hospital. Journal of Psychosocial Nursing, 37(11), 35-39.

Gordon, M. (1997). Manual of nursing diagnoses 1997-1998 edition. St. Louis: Mosby.

Grady, P. A. (2000). News from NINR. Nursing Outlook, 48(1) 33.

Guyton, A. C. & Hall, J. E. (1995). Textbook of medical physiology (9th ed.). Philadelphia: Saunders.

Hajagos, K., Geiser, P., Parker, B., & Tesfa, A. (1998). Safer-sex education for persons with mental illness. Journal of Psychosocial Nursing and Mental Health Services, 36(8), 33-37.

Hewlett, P., & Eichelberger, L. (1996). The case against mandatory continuing education. Journal of Continuing Education in Nursing, 27(4), 176-181.

Hinshaw, A. S., Feetham, S. L., Shaver, J. L. (1999). Handbook of clinical nursing research. Thousand Oaks, CA: Sage.

Holm, K., & Llewellyn, J. G. (1986). Nursing research for nursing practice. Philadelphia: Saunders.

Jennings, B. M. & Staggers, N. (1999). A provocative look at performance measurement. Nursing Administration Quarterly, 24(1), 17-30.

Johnson, M., Maas, M., & Moorhead, S. (Eds.). (1999). Nursing outcomes classification (NOC). St. Louis: Mosby.

Leininger, M. (1994). Transcultural nursing: Concepts, theories, and practices. Columbus, OH: Greyden Press.

Levine, M. (1995). The rhetoric of nursing theory. Image: Journal of Nursing Scholarship. 27(1), 14.

Lindeman, C. A. (2000). The future of nursing education. Journal of Nursing Education, 39(1), 5-12.

Masching, J. (1996). A nurse battling with her own depression. Journal of Psychosocial Nursing, 34(9), 26-29.

McKibbin, R. C., Brimmer, P. F., Clinton, J. F., & Galliher, J. M. (1985). DRGs and nursing care. Kansas City: American Nurses Association.

Meleis, A. (1991). Theoretical nursing: Development and progress (2nd ed.). Philadelphia: Lippincott.

Moss, M. T. (1995). Perioperative nursing in the managed care era: Foundations of nursing empowerment. Nursing Economics, 13(2), 112-114.

Neil, J., & Barrell, L. (1998). Transition theory and its relevance to patients with chronic wounds. Rehabilitation Nurse, 23(6), 295-299.

Newman, M. (1986). Health as expanding consciousness. St. Louis: Mosby.

Norwood, B. R. (1997). The nursing process. In K. K. Chitty, (Ed.), Professional nursing: Concepts and challenges (2nd ed.). Philadelphia: W. B. Saunders.

Oermann, M. H., & Huber, D. (1999). Patient outcomes: A measure of nursing's value. American Journal of Nursing, 99(9), 40-47.

Orem, D. E. (1995). Nursing: Concepts of practice. (5th ed.). St. Louis: Mosby.

Parse, R. (1987). Nursing science: Major paradigms, theories, and critiques. Philadelphia: Saunders.

Peplau, H. (1952). Interpersonal relations in nursing. New York: Putnam.

Peplau, H. (1960). Talking with patients. American Journal of Nursing, 60(7), 964.

Pesut, D. J., & Herman, J. (1999). Clinical reasoning: The art and science of critical and creative thinking. Albany, NY: Delmar Publishers.

Pesut, D., & Herman, J. (1999). Clinical reasoning: The art and science of critical and creative thinking. Albany, NY: Delmar Publishers.

Polk, L. (1997). Toward a middle-range theory of resilience. Advances in Nursing Science, 19(3), 1-13.

Roberts, B., Madigan, E., Anthony, M., & Pabst, S. (1996). The congruence of nursing diagnoses and supporting clinical evidence. Nursing Diagnosis, 7(3), 108-115.

Rogers, M. (1970). An introduction to the theoretical basis of nursing. Philadelphia: F. A. Davis.

Roy, C., & Andrews, H. A. (1991). The Roy Adaptation Model: The definitive statement. Norwalk, CT: Appleton & Lange.

Ruesch, J. (1961). Therapeutic communication. New York: Norton.

Schaff, A. W. (1990). Meditations for women who do too much. New York: HarperCollins.

Sparks, S. M., & Taylor, C. M. (1995). Nursing diagnosis reference manual (3rd ed.). Springhouse, PA: Springhouse.

Sparks, S., & Taylor, C. (1994). Formulating a nursing diagnosis. Nursing94, 24(3), 32H, 32J.

Stratton, T. D., Dunkin, J. W., & Juhl, N. (1995). Redefining the nursing shortage: A rural perspective. Nursing Outlook, 43(2), 71-77.

Stuart, G., & Laraia, M. (1998). Stuart & Sundeen's principles and practice of psychiatric nursing (6th ed.). St. Louis: Mosby.

Tschikota, S. (1993). The clinical decision-making processes of student nurses. Journal of Nursing Education, 32(9), 389-405.

Varcarolis, E., & Rader, I. (1998). Foundations of mental health-psychiatric nursing (3rd ed.). Philadelphia: Saunders.

Wachtel, P. (1993). Principles of therapeutic communication. New York: Guilford Press.

Watson, J. (1985). Nursing: Human science and human care. Norwalk, CT: Appleton-Century-Crofts.

Whitley, G. (1999). Processes and methodologies for research validation of nursing diagnoses. Nursing Diagnosis, 10(1), 5-13.

Index

O

P

R

S